Optometry 101

Differential Diagnosis of Ocular Diseases

Tahiba Begum
BSc (Hons) MCOptom

Copyright © 2022 by Tahiba Begum. All rights reserved.
Cover designer: Muhammad Junaid

The right of Tahiba Begum identified as the author of this book, asserted by her in accordance with the Copyright, Designs and Patents Act 1988.

No part of this publication may be reproduced, distributed, or transmitted in any form or by any means, electronic or mechanical, including photocopying, or any information storage and retrieval system, without permission in writing from the author, except for non-commercial uses permitted by UK copyright law. Copying, re-publishing, or redistributing is prohibited and will constitute an infringement of copyright and theft of the author's intellectual property. For details on how to seek permission or to give feedback, please contact **optometry101@outlook.com**

ISBN: 978-1-3999-3851-8

NOTICE

Our principal aim is to provide a clear understanding of Optometry in everyday practice to undergraduate students in their final year of studies, pre-registration students and any practitioner wishing to review their clinical knowledge or returning to work following a leave of absence. The intended purpose of this book is to be a guide only, and any intended user should exercise their judgement and expertise when dealing with patients on a case-by-case basis.

This book was published in November 2022. The user should be aware of any updates, significant developments and advancements in the medical sciences and world of Optometry beyond this point. To the fullest extent of the law, no responsibility is assumed by the author for any injury and/ or damage to persons or property as a matter of product liability, negligence or otherwise, contained in the material therein.

LIST OF CONTRIBUTORS

My deepest gratitude to the individuals who reviewed and edited Optometry 101, Differential Diagnosis in preparation for publication:

Tahrima Hurany Begum BSc (Hons) Optometry
Arfah Ali BScOptom
Thaslima Begum BScOptom
Iram Arshad BScOptom
Bushra Chaudri BSc (Hons) Optometry
Mohammed Joyenal Bashar
Loshima Begum LLB (Hons), Solicitor
Nurany Ryhan BA (Hons) Primary Education, Teacher

"In the name of Allah, the most merciful and compassionate."

I thank Allah for the countless blessings in my life, my children and the inspirational people who have supported me during this journey.

'May this book be a means for you to benefit long term, and may it be sadaqah jariyah for me. May Allah grant you beneficial knowledge and the ability to act upon it.'

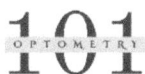

TABLE OF CONTENT

Chapters 1: Referral Guidelines   6-7

Chapter 2: Signs, Symptoms And Differential Diagnosis
- **2.1** Headache   8-9
- **2.2** A gradual decrease in vision   10-11
- **2.3** A painless, sudden decrease in vision   12-13
- **2.4** A painful, sudden decrease in vision   14-15
- **2.5** Diplopia   16-17
- **2.6** Red eye: mildly painful or asymptomatic   18
- **2.7** Severe painful red eye   19-20
- **2.8** Optic disc oedema   21-22
- **2.9** Abnormal pupils   23-24
- **2.10** Is the lesion cancerous?   25

Chapter 3: How To Differentiate…
- **3.1** Cataract   26-27
- **3.2** Glaucoma   28-30
- **3.3** Diabetic Retinopathy   31
- **3.4** Diabetic Maculopathy   32
- **3.5** Hypertensive Retinopathy   33-34
- **3.6** Macular Degeneration   35-36
- **3.7** Vitreous Detachment   37-38
- **3.8** Retinal Detachment   39-40
- **3.9** Vascular Occlusions   41-43
- **3.10** Optic Neuropathy vs Optic Neuritis   44-45
- **3.11** Uveitis   46-47
- **3.12** Blepharitis   48-49
- **3.13** Conjunctivitis   50-53
- **3.14** Disorders of the conjunctiva and sclera   54-56
- **3.15** Contact lens associated infiltrative keratitis   57-59

Chapter 4: Binocular Vision Abnormalities
- **4.1** Muscle inaction   60
- **4.2** Incomitance   61-62

Chapter 5: Accurate Recording And Analysis
- **5.1** H&S sight test   63-65
- **5.2** Referral letter template   66
- **5.3** H&S contact lens aftercare   67
- **5.4** CLs tests and appropriate recording   68-70
- **5.5** Visual field analysis   71
- **5.6** Where in the visual pathway?   72-73

Abbreviations   75
Bibliography   76-78

REFERRAL GUIDELINES

There will always be minor differences in the referral protocol depending on locality and area of work. For this reason, please use the table below as a guide but always refer to the local referral guidelines.

Emergency (ASAP)	Emergency (Within 24 Hours)	Urgent (Call HES to triage)	Routine
Sudden, complete loss of vision <6 hours	Sudden, unknown cause of vision loss (< 24h)	Sudden change in vision < 2/52	Cataract
Retinal Artery Occlusion <12hrs	Papilloedema	CRVO with elevated IOP (< 40mmHg)	Open Angle Glaucoma
Acute Angle Closure Glaucoma	Malignant Hypertensive Retinopathy	BRVO + central foveal haemorrhage	Background and Pre-proliferative Diabetic Retinopathy
Severe eye pain with nausea or vomiting	Pain on ocular movement	Amaurosis fugax: refer to the GP for a TIA work-up	Diabetic Maculopathy
Endophthalmitis	IOP ≥ 40mmHg	IOP > 35mmHg	Dry AMD
Retinal Detachment: Macula on	RD: Macula off	Proliferative Diabetic Retinopathy	Macula Hole
Suspected Giant Cell Arteritis	Symptomatic retinal tears, holes & breaks	Iris Rubeosis	Pterygium
RAPD	Floaters/ photopsia < 48 hrs + tobacco dust	New pupillary defects	Keratoconus
Acute onset of: Diplopia Squint Ptosis	PVD-related vitreous haemorrhage	Vitreous haemorrhage (non-PVD)	
Acute Proptosis	Uveitis/ Iritis	Wet AMD	
Nerve palsy (new, sudden, or worse)	Scleritis	Myopic CNV	
Chemical trauma	Hypopyon	Marginal Keratitis	
Blunt trauma	Infective Keratitis	Atopic Keratoconjuctivitis Vernal Keratoconjuctivitis	
	Herpetic infection (Simplex/ Zoster)	Central Serous Retinopathy	
	Traumatic Red Eye	Optic Neuritis	

This list is not exhaustive. Optometrists should always apply their clinical judgment when deciding on the appropriate clinical management.

ADDITIONAL NOTES

SIGNS, SYMPTOMS AND DIFFERENTIAL DIAGNOSIS

Ocular conditions are categorised by their presenting symptoms and ocular signs. This chapter will help in narrowing the options for an accurate diagnosis. The Optometrist may observe some/ all of the signs and symptoms mentioned for each condition; however, this list is not exhaustive, and one should always apply their clinical judgment when dealing with patients on a case-by-case basis. Once a tentative diagnosis has been made, refer to the designated area in chapter three for further details of the ocular condition.

2.1 HEADACHE

1. **Asthenia**
   Cause: Uncorrected refractive error, presbyopia, decompensating phoria, excessive use of VDU etc.
   Symptoms: Frontal headache and eyestrain (worse at the end of the day or task specific).
2. **Migraine**
   Symptoms: Moderate to severe headache, throbbing pain, usually on one side of the head (the episode can last for hours to several days), feeling sick and increased sensitivity to light and sound. In addition, certain triggers exacerbate symptoms, e.g. stress, sleeping pattern and hormonal levels.
3. **Migraine with aura**
   The patient may report a small ball-like appearance or visual disturbance that enlarges and extends to obstruct vision. The episode can last up to 45 minutes.
   Symptoms: Numbness, a change in taste and smell, with or without a migraine headache, but usually precedes a headache (sitting in a dark room reduces the symptoms).
   In all sub-categories of a migraine, there will be no floaters, shadows, 'curtain over vision' or any risk factor suggesting this is a Retinal Detachment.
4. **Binocular Vision abnormalities**
   Symptoms: Frontal headache, intermittent blur, eye strain and diplopia.
   (These symptoms can intensify when tired, stressed or can be task-specific).
   Signs: Binocular amp of accom (AA) < monocular AA, slip in mallet unit, NPC >10cm, breakdown of a phoria and poor recovery. Signs and symptoms depend on the cause of the binocular vision abnormality; therefore, this list is not exhaustive.
5. **Raised Intracranial Pressure**
   Symptoms: Constant headache, transient loss of vision (lasting a few seconds), sudden onset of diplopia, feeling sleepy, unwell, vomiting (often projectile) and a throbbing sensation often described as a 'whooshing sound.' The headache exacerbates in the morning, with head movements, coughing and straining.
   Signs: Usually bilateral, asymmetrical, pupillary changes, and an enlarged blind spot. Examination reveals papilloedema consisting of severe disc hyperaemia, blurred disc margins and disc elevation without a physiological cup.
6. **Acute Closed Angle Glaucoma**
   Symptoms: Halos around lights, transient blurred vision (can be reported as 'misty vision'), ipsilateral frontal headache, severe eye pain (ache around the eye) and nausea.
   Signs: Fixed mid-dilated pupil (oval and unresponsive to light), raised IOP (>40mmHg), narrow/ closed anterior chamber angles, hypermetropia (positive shift in Rx), circumlimbal injection, corneal oedema, anterior cells and flare, normal disc or disc oedema with venous congestion and haemorrhages.

7. **Malignant Hypertensive Retinopathy**
   Symptoms: Severe headache, variable loss of vision, nausea, and vomiting.
   Signs: Macula star (a ring of exudates from the disc to the macula), disc oedema, arterial narrowing, haemorrhages, cotton wool spots and exudates. Signs of Non-Malignant Hypertensive Retinopathy will also be present, e.g. arteriolar tortuosity, arteriosclerosis.
8. **Optic Neuritis**
   Symptoms: Pain with eye movement in extreme gazes, eye and brow pain, blurred vision, impaired night vision, red desaturation (colour appears washed out), and impaired depth perception (difficult to judge distances when walking up and down stairs etc.)
   Signs: Central VA and visual field loss, RAPD (if unilateral), reduction in contrast sensitivity, and optic nerve swelling (Papillitis or Neuroretinitis).
9. **Giant Cell Arteritis associated AION**
   Symptoms: Headache (frontal/ temporal/ occipital/ generalised) exacerbates when lying down, jaw pain or pain whilst chewing, periocular pain, scalp tenderness and the patient may feel unwell.
   Signs: Sudden severe VA loss, RAPD, swollen 'chalky white' discs with splinter or flame-shaped haemorrhages.
10. **Uveitis**
    Symptoms: Pain, a red eye, and photophobia.
    Signs: Intraocular inflammation (depending on the area affected), pupillary changes, cells and flare. This condition is subdivided into multiple categories. For further details, refer to 'Chapter 3, Uveitis.'
11. **Pituitary Melanoma**
    Symptoms: Headache is worse on waking.
    Signs: Visual field defect (bitemporal hemianopia or upper temporal quadranopia).

This list is not exhaustive.

Important Gems: Recommended Tests
Headache: Visual field test, OCT, colour vision test, ocular motility, pupil assessment and anterior chamber assessment (Van Herricks).

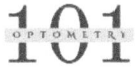

2.2 A GRADUAL DECREASE IN VISION

1. **Refractive error (RE):** myopia, astigmatism etc.
   Symptoms: Reduced vision with current spectacles/ patient reports wearing out-of-date spectacles or not wearing their spectacles at all.
   Signs: The pinhole test improves VA, and there is a refractive change in Rx.
2. **Cataract**
   Symptoms: Vision affected by lighting conditions and glare.
   Signs: Reduced VA and visual field (area affected depends on the type of Cataract present).
   Cortical cataract: Wedge-shaped or radial spoke-like opacity.
   Nuclear Sclerotic Cataract: Yellowing and brunescence of the crystalline lens.
   PSC: Vacuolated or granular-like appearance. (For details, refer to 'Chapter 3, Cataract.')
3. **Open Angle Glaucoma**
   No/ minimal symptoms reported until the disease has advanced, e.g. tunnel vision.
   Signs
   - Raised IOP: >24mmHg.
   - Open anterior chamber angles.
   - Optic nerve head damage: Asymmetry in the CD ratio (>0.2 between the two eyes), large CD ratio (>0.6), vertical elongation of the cup (oval-shaped), cupping and ISNT rule NOT followed.
   - Vascular clinical changes: A nasal shift of disc vessels, baring, bayonetting with or without splinter haemorrhages.
   - VF defect: paracentral scotoma, arcuate scotoma, nasal step, temporal wedges etc.
4. **Dry Age Related Macular Degeneration**
   Symptoms: Difficulty recognising faces & reading. In some cases, patients are asymptomatic.
   Signs: Central VA loss, positive scotoma on Amsler, examination reveals drusen (hard or soft), RPE degeneration, which includes a variable amount of hyper/ hypopigmentation and atrophy of the RPE, which can eventually lead to geographic atrophy of the RPE (last stage).
5. **Diabetic Retinopathy**
   Subdivided into Background, Pre-proliferative and Proliferative Diabetic Retinopathy.
   Signs: For details, refer to 'Chapter 3, Diabetic Retinopathy'.
6. **Diabetic Maculopathy**
   Must have clinically significant signs to be categorised as Diabetic Maculopathy. This includes any exudates within 1DD of the centre of the fovea, a group of exudates within the macula area, any microaneurysms/ haemorrhages within 1DD of the macula with VA < 6/12.
7. **Posterior Capsular Opacification**
   Symptoms: Gradual decrease in vision (hazy, cloudy, blurred), glare and monocular diplopia. The patient reports similar symptoms to those previously raised before cataract surgery.
   Signs: Reduced VA, vacuolated appearance, 'elschnig pearls,' difficulty viewing fundus due to the PCO, a dull reflex seen on retinoscopy and reduced contrast sensitivity. There are multiple patterns of opacification, each unique in appearance, e.g. fibrosis-type PCO.
8. **Keratoconus**
   Symptoms: Vision appears reduced despite up-to-date spectacles given, excessive eye rubbing and monocular diplopia.
   Signs: Frequent change in spectacles, oblique and irregular astigmatism, myopic shift, scissor reflex & distortion on retinoscopy, oil droplet reflex in ophthalmoscopy, Vogt striae, corneal scarring, a conical appearance to the cornea, Fleischer's ring and Munson sign (latter stage).
9. **Cone Dystrophy**
   Symptoms: Photophobia and loss of detailed vision (symptoms can vary massively).
   Signs: Central VA loss, colour vision affected (usually deutan-tritan defect) and nystagmus can also develop. The macula may appear normal or show pigmentary changes, bull's eye maculopathy, RPE atrophy and geographic atrophy.

10. **Corneal Dystrophy**
    Subdivided into Epithelial, Stromal and Endothelial Corneal Dystrophy.
    Symptoms: Photophobia, glare and pain (ranging from discomfort, a foreign body sensation to severe dry eye). In some cases, the patient is asymptomatic.
    Signs: Usually a bilateral, non-inflammatory, non-infectious opacifying condition.
    (The signs observed will depend on the cause and area affected)

11. **Anterior Scleritis**
    Subdivided into non-necrotizing and necrotizing with inflammation.
    Symptoms: Deep pain (orbit, eyebrow, jaw, temple), tenderness of the globe, watery eyes and photophobia.
    Signs: Injection of scleral, episcleral and conjunctival vessels.

Anterior Non-necrotizing Scleritis
   Usually unilateral, either diffuse or nodular in appearance (scleral nodules do not move over the underlying tissue).
   ❖ Diffuse
   Symptoms: Ocular discomfort progressing to aches and pains to the temple and face (worse in the morning but can improve throughout the day).
   Signs: Generalised redness or local to one quadrant.
   ❖ Nodular
   Symptoms: A gradual onset of pain, redness and tenderness of the globe.
   Signs: Scleral nodules that are bluish-red and immobile.

Anterior Necrotizing with Inflammation
   Usually bilateral, pain can be minimal but VA loss is severe (poor prognosis of recovery).
   Symptoms: A gradual increase in pain, which can extend to the brow, jaw and temple.
   Signs: This can vary depending on the cause; however, the sclera is affected in all cases.

---

12. **Transient loss due to Amaurosis Fugax**
    Symptoms: Temporary loss of vision reported as 'clouding over,' lasts for seconds-minutes.
    Signs: Can be linked to Central Retinal Artery Occlusion. For details, refer to 'Chapter 3, Occlusions'.

This list is not exhaustive.

Important Gems: Recommended Tests
Reduced Vision: Visual acuity assessment, pinhole test, amsler test, contrast sensitivity test, visual field test, OCT, pupil assessment and anterior chamber assessment (Van Herricks).

2.3 PAINLESS, SUDDEN DECREASE IN VISION

1. **Proliferative Diabetic Retinopathy**
   Symptoms: Blurry and/ or fluctuating vision.
   Signs: Neovascularisation including NVD (1/3DD) or NVE (1/2DD), pre-retinal or vitreous haemorrhage, rubeosis iridis and signs of Background and Pre-proliferative DR are also visible in all four quadrants (IRMA, haemorrhages, venous and arterial changes etc.)
2. **Retinal Detachment**
   Subdivided into Rhegmatogenous, Tractional and Exudative Retinal Detachment.
   Symptoms: Flashes (photopsia), floaters, shadows or 'curtain in their vision.'
   Signs: Sudden decrease in VA and visual field (if the macula is involved), tobacco dust, lower IOP in the affected eye (can be 5mmHg lower), a RAPD can occur when the macula or two quadrants of the retina is detached, retinal tears, breaks or holes, macula on/ off and may have vitreoretinal degeneration (lattice degeneration etc.)
3. **Central Serous Retinopathy**
   Symptoms: Unilateral blurred vision, objects appearing smaller (micropsia), metamorphopsia and mild dyschromatopsia.
   Signs: VA (6/9-6/18), round or oval serous detachment at the macula, positive scotoma, and decreased contrast sensitivity.
4. **Non-arteritic Ischaemic Optic Neuropathy (NAION)**
   Symptoms: Reduced vision in the affected eye (within hours to days of initial onset or sudden decrease upon waking) and dyschromatopsia.
   Signs: Disc oedema with or without splinter haemorrhages, altitudinal visual field defect (commonly an inferior defect causing an absolute scotoma, but can also be a central, paracentral or arcuate defect).
5. **Occlusions: CRAO and CRVO**

CRAO
Symptoms: Unilateral ring of blindness that progresses inwards from the periphery towards the centre, can take two hours to progress or notice upon waking. This can be seen as a complete/ transient loss of vision or vision that resolves spontaneously.
Signs: Reduced visual acuity (6/60 or less), RAPD in the affected eye, disc oedema, cherry red spot at the macula, the fundus is cloudy or yellow, and arteries are the same colour and thickness as veins.
> **Relevant Tests**: Monocular VA testing, pupil assessment, visual field testing (if suspicious of BRAO) and a dilated fundus examination.

CRVO
Subdivided into Ischaemic and Non-ischaemic Central Retinal Vein Occlusion.
1. **Non-ischaemic CRVO**
   Symptoms: Sudden unilateral loss of vision or blurred vision. In some cases, the patient is asymptomatic.
   Signs: Variable VA (ranges from 6/6-CF), RAPD is mild or absent, retinal and disc oedema, cotton wool spots, haemorrhage (superficial, deep blot and flame-shaped), IRMA, dilated and tortuous veins.
2. **Ischaemic CRVO**
   Symptoms: Sudden and severe reduction in vision often noticed upon waking.
   Signs: Variable VA (CF or worse), marked RAPD, disc and macula oedema, cotton wool spots, haemorrhage (superficial, deep blot, flame-shaped), IRMA, dilated and tortuous veins.

These signs may obscure the fundus view and are present in all four quadrants.

6. **Wet AMD**
   Symptoms: Sudden onset of distorted monocular vision (straight lines appear wavy or crooked) and positive scotoma (if haemorrhages are present).
   Signs: Hyperopic shift, choroidal neo-vascularisation (green, grey or pinkish yellow), exudated serous and blood near the macula (red if subretinal, darker if sub-RPE) and a disciform scar (latter stage).
7. **Macular Hole**
   Symptoms: Central vision affected with or without metamorphopsia. In some cases, the patient is asymptomatic.
   Signs: Yellow or white lesion at the macula. The size and shape of the hole can vary (ring, crescent-shaped etc.)

This list is not exhaustive.

Important Gems: Recommended Tests
Macula Abnormalities:
1. Amsler: Look for metamorphopsia (distortion) or scotoma (missing areas). Relevant question: 'Looking at the central dot, do you see any wavy, missing or broken lines?'
2. Photostress recovery test: Shine a light on the eye for 10 seconds and time the recovery (in seconds) for the patient to see one line above their best-corrected visual acuity. (Normal < 60 seconds)
3. Maddox rod: The patient may report a break or distortion in the image. This will help distinguish between distortion and central suppression.
4. Pinhole: Same or worse VA observed.
5. Additional tests recommended: Visual field test, colour vision test and pupil assessment.

2.4 PAINFUL, SUDDEN DECREASE IN VISION

1. **Closed Angle Glaucoma**
   Symptoms: Halos around lights, transient blurred vision (can be reported as 'misty vision'), ipsilateral frontal headache, severe eye pain (ache around the eye) and nausea.
   Signs: Fixed mid-dilated pupil (oval and unresponsive to light), raised IOP (>40mmHg), narrow/ closed anterior chamber angles, hypermetropia (positive shift in Rx), circumlimbal injection, corneal oedema, anterior cells and flare, normal disc or disc oedema with venous congestion and haemorrhages.
2. **Malignant Hypertensive Retinopathy**
   Symptoms: Severe headache, variable loss of vision, nausea and vomiting.
   Signs: Macula star, disc oedema, arterial narrowing, haemorrhages, cotton wool spots and exudates. Signs of Non-Malignant Hypertensive Retinopathy will also be present, e.g. arteriolar tortuosity, arteriosclerosis.
3. **Corneal Ulcer**
   Symptoms: Photophobia, teary eyes and a red eye.
   Signs: Ulcer (large if >2mm), grey or white, dot-like appearance but can vary depending on the cause, epithelium and/or stromal stain with fluorescein (fuzzy edges), conjunctival redness, ptosis, lid swelling, discharge, anterior chamber activity (cells & flare) and a reduction in the visual acuity (if the ulcer is close to the visual axis).
4. **Keratitis**
   Multiple aetiology, photophobia reported and ulcer/ infiltrate observed (shape and size vary). Common examples of Microbial Keratitis are below:

Bacterial Keratitis
Symptoms: Photophobia, blurred vision and purulent/ mucopurulent discharge.
Signs: Variable signs depending on the severity and cause of the condition.
Ranges from infiltrates causing an epithelial defect, stromal oedema and eyelid swelling to scarring, ulceration and secondary conditions such as Anterior Uveitis, Endophthalmitis etc.

Herpes Simplex Keratitis
Symptoms: Variable symptoms include pain (burning, irritation), lacrimation and/or reports of a recurrent cold sore (Optometrist may see a cold sore on examination).
Signs: Dendritic ulcer/s, keratic precipitates (KP), secondary conditions such as Uveitis and reduced contrast sensitivity.
If not treated appropriately, this can lead to a geographic/ amoebic ulcer.

Herpes Zoster ophthalmicus
Symptoms: Discomfort and teary eyes (lacrimation).
Signs: Variable with different severities. Hutchinson's sign (a lesion on the tip of the nose). Keratitis amongst many other secondary conditions is observed on examination.

Protozoa: Acanthamoeba Keratitis
May have mild signs, but symptoms are severe.
Symptoms: Usually unilateral, moderate to severe eye pain (difficulty opening their eyes), photophobia and no relief even after contact lens removal. The patient may report poor contact lens hygiene, recent corneal trauma or water exposure (swims or showers with lenses and cleans lenses/ case with tap water).
Signs: Large ulcer and reduced VA (at least a two-line reduction in the Snellen chart).
This condition can be difficult to diagnose. In the initial stages, the signs are mild and may resemble Viral Conjunctivitis, but then it can appear like Herpes Simplex Keratitis. If still not managed accordingly, it can progress to stromal penetration with cells, flare and hypopyon.

5. **Acute Anterior Uveitis**
   Symptoms: Photophobia, dull aching pain (worse when reading/ accommodating), a red eye, teary eyes (lacrimation) and the patient may report episodes of ocular discomfort a few days before the acute attack.
   Signs: Variable VA (poor VA when there is severe hypopyon), miotic or sluggish pupil, circumcorneal injection, posterior synechiae, cells and flare in the anterior chamber, iris nodules (Koeppe/ Busacca) and keratic precipitates.
6. **Giant Cell Arteritis associated AION**
   Symptoms: Headache (frontal/ temporal/ occipital/ generalised) exacerbates when lying down, jaw pain or pain whilst chewing, periocular pain, scalp tenderness and the patient may feel unwell.
   Signs: Sudden severe VA loss, RAPD, swollen 'chalky white' discs with splinter or flame-shaped haemorrhages. For further details, refer to 'Chapter 3, Optic Neuropathy VS Optic Neuritis'
7. **Bacterial Orbital Cellulitis (severe sight and life-threatening)**
   Symptoms: Severely tender and sore lids, a painful red eye which is worse with eye movement, headache, reduced vision, double vision, fever (recent upper respiratory symptoms e.g. nasal discharge)
   Signs: Ptosis, oedematous lids, proptosis, reduced VA and possible impaired colour. RAPD and optic nerve involvement (in severe cases).
   (Signs are usually unilateral but oedema can occur in the other eye).

This list is not exhaustive.

2.5 DIPLOPIA

Monocular Diplopia
1. **Uncorrected Astigmatism**
   Symptoms: Headache, eye strain, distorted or blurry vision.
2. **Cortical Cataract**
   Symptoms: Difficulty reading (worse in dim light), glare whilst driving at night and diplopia (usually in the early stages of the condition).
   Signs: Wedge-shaped spokes found in the periphery of the crystalline lens, Rx change, astigmatic change, reduced contrast sensitivity and sector loss in the visual field.
3. **Posterior Capsular Opacification**
   Symptoms: A gradual decrease in vision (hazy, cloudy or blurred) and glare. The patient reports similar symptoms to those previously raised before cataract surgery.
   Signs: 'Elschnig pearls,' vacuolated appearance, a dull retinoscopy reflex, reduced VA and contrast sensitivity. There are multiple patterns of opacification, each unique in appearance, e.g. fibrosis-type PCO.
4. **Corneal irregularity, e.g. Keratoconus**
   Symptoms: Vision appears reduced despite up-to-date Rx given and excessive eye rubbing.
   Signs: Frequent but gradual change in Rx, oblique and irregular astigmatism, myopic shift, scissor reflex/ distortion on retinoscopy, oil droplet reflex in ophthalmoscopy, Vogt striae, corneal scarring, a conical appearance to the cornea, Fleischer's ring and Munson sign.
5. **Medications,** e.g. antidepressants, antihistamines.
   This can cause dryness of the ocular surface/ tear film instability, which can induce diplopia.

Binocular Diplopia
1. **Binocular Vision abnormalities**
   Symptoms: Frontal headache, intermittent blur and eye strain.
   (These symptoms can intensify when tired, stressed or can be task-specific).
   Signs: Break down of a phoria, poor recovery, slip in mallet unit, NPC >10cm, binocular amp of accom (AA) < monocular AA. Signs and symptoms depend on the cause of the binocular vision abnormality; therefore, this list is not exhaustive.
   Convergence Insufficiency
   Symptoms: Headache and tension in and around the eye (eye strain), blurred vision and the patient may complain of frequent loss of place when reading.
   Signs: Low AC/A, reduced near point of convergence and positive fusional vergence etc.
   Decompensating Phoria
   Symptoms: Frontal headache, intermittent blurred vision and diplopia commonly reported at near. These symptoms can intensify when the patient is stressed, fatigued or unwell.
   Management: Orthoptic exercises, and if the patient has a decompensating exophoria, prescribe base-in prisms and negative Rx.
2. **Induced prismatic effect due to spectacle prescription**
   Symptoms: Blurred vision, asthenopia and headache.
   Signs: Poorly fitted spectacles (not looking through the optical centre of the lens etc.)
3. **Direct Trauma to the Eye**
   If the orbital wall fractures, this can cause EOM entrapment or mechanical restriction.
4. **Diplopia due to Other Causes**
   - Thyroid Eye Disease: Graves Disease causing vertical diplopia.
   - Myasthenia Gravis: Ptosis (usually unilateral), EOM palsies and incomitant strabismus (worse at the end of the day/ fatigue but can improve with rest).
   - Parkinson's Disease: Can cause convergence insufficiency resulting in diplopia and manifesting as an exotropia that is worse at near.
   - Additional causes: Tumour, Cellulitis, Temporal Arteritis, Scleritis etc.

Sudden Onset Diplopia

1. **Nerve Palsy**
   Symptoms: Difficulty looking towards a particular position of gaze.
   Signs: Abnormal head posture (face turn/ chin elevation or depression/ head tilt). Signs and symptoms vary depending on if the condition is recently acquired or is longstanding.
   Signs of incomitancy: A sudden onset of diplopia, headache and pupil involvement.

   Sixth Nerve Palsy   **EOM: (Lateral Rectus affected)**
   Cause: Multiple Sclerosis, Diabetes, hypertension, trauma etc.
   Signs: Esotropia in the primary position (cannot move the eye to the temporal side; therefore, the primary position is affected, and the eye turns **in**).
   For long-standing sixth nerve palsies: There is a limitation of abduction with normal adduction of the affected eye. This is more obvious when looking at a distant target and less obvious/ minimal for near targets.

   Fourth Nerve Palsy   **(Superior Oblique affected)**
   Cause: Trauma, congenital, microvascular disease or idiopathic
   Signs: Ipsilateral hypertropia and excyclotorsion. May develop a head tilt.

   Third Nerve Palsy   **(SR, MR, IR, IO affected)**
   Cause: Diabetes, hypertension, tumour, trauma etc.
   Symptoms: Reports of tilting the head to either reduce diplopia or separate the double images so that it is easier to distinguish them.
   Signs: Eye is **down and out,** ptosis, mydriasis, loss of pupil action (fixed, dilated pupils) and paresis of accommodation.

2. **Aneurysm of the Posterior Communicating Artery**
   Symptoms: Asymptomatic or severe headache, vision is affected, and cranial nerve deficit.
   Signs: Heteronymous (bi-nasal) visual field defect.
3. **Microvascular/ Raised Intracranial Pressure**
   Symptoms: Constant headache, transient loss of vision (lasting a few seconds), feeling sleepy, unwell, vomiting (often projectile) and a throbbing sensation described as a 'whooshing sound.' The headache exacerbates in the morning, with head movements, coughing or straining.
   Signs: Usually bilateral, asymmetrical, pupillary changes and an enlarged blind spot. Fundus examination reveals papilloedema consisting of severe disc hyperaemia, blurred disc margins and disc elevation without a physiological cup.
4. **Posterior Scleritis**
   Symptoms: Severe reduction in vision and painful restriction of eye movements.
   Signs: Ptosis, proptosis, disc oedema with or without cotton wool spots, macula oedema, exudative retinal detachment and choroidal folds. Signs and symptoms of Anterior Scleritis can be observed too. In some cases, the patient may present with no obvious abnormalities, e.g. serious symptoms but quiet white eyes.
5. **Head Trauma/ Direct Trauma to the Eye**
   Symptoms: Ranges from blurred vision to complete loss of central and peripheral vision. May also report symptoms of a concussion.
   Signs and symptoms are variable and depend on the severity of the injury.

Important Gems: Recommended Tests
Diplopia: Ocular motility, cover test, fixation disparity tests, visual field test and pupil assessment.
Binocular Diplopia: Diplopia will disappear when one eye is covered and can be mechanical or neurological.

2.6 RED EYE: MILDLY PAINFUL/ASYMPTOMATIC

1. **Blepharitis**
   Symptoms: Ocular discomfort (burning, gritty, foreign body sensation), sore or itchy lids, mild photophobia, blurred vision, contact lens intolerance, and the patient may report symptoms similar to dry eye. In some cases, the patient is asymptomatic.
   Signs: Usually bilateral, lids are red and inflamed, eyelashes appear misdirected, missing, trichinosis, madarosis, crustiness and white scales on the roots, conjunctival hyperaemia and recurrent styes.

2. **Conjunctivitis**
   Subdivided into Infective, Allergic, Traumatic and Systemic.
   Differentiate the different types of Conjunctivitis by its discharge.
   - ❖ Muco-purulent discharge: Mild Bacterial or Chlamydial Conjunctivitis.
   - ❖ Mucous: Vernal Conjunctivitis.
   - ❖ Purulent: Bacterial Conjunctivitis.
   - ❖ Watery: Viral and Allergic (acute) Conjunctivitis.

   Common forms of Conjunctivitis and their distinguishing features are described below:

Infected
- **Bacterial Conjunctivitis**
  Symptoms: FB sensation, sore and gritty eyes, and eyelids stuck together upon waking.
  Signs: Purulent/ mucopurulent discharge, lid crusting, conjunctival hyperaemia and mild papillary reaction at the tarsal conjunctiva.
- **Viral Conjunctivitis**
  Symptoms: mild burning sensation and flu-like symptoms.
  Signs: Watery discharge, tender pre-auricular lymph nodes, fine papillae, and follicles can be present at the tarsal conjunctiva and/or lower fornix.

Allergic
- **Seasonal Allergic Conjunctivitis**
  Symptoms: Itchy eyes, sneezing and nasal discharge. These symptoms are seasonal.
  Signs: A watery or mucous discharge, no pre-auricular lymph node swelling, mild/ moderate oedema, and hyperaemia of the bulbar and tarsal conjunctiva with a papillary reaction.
- **Perennial Allergic Conjunctivitis**
  Symptoms and signs are similar to SAC but can occur all year round.
  To note: The cornea will not be affected in both cases.

Traumatic
- **Giant Papillary Conjunctivitis (GPC)**
  Symptoms: Itchy eyes (may increase after lens removal), blurred vision, decreased comfort and lens intolerance.
  Signs: Bilateral condition but asymmetrical depending on the cause of the trauma.
  Reduced VA (if there is stringy mucous discharge), upper tarsal conjunctiva usually affected, papillae (macropapillae/ giant papillae), conjunctival oedema and conjunctival hyperaemia.

---

3. **Episcleritis**
   Symptoms: Mild pain (ache/ burning sensation) and photophobia.
   Signs: Sectoral hyperaemic injection with/ without nodules (diffused or in one area).

4. **Subconjunctival Haemorrhage**
   Symptoms: Spontaneous redness with no report of pain, swelling or reduced vision.
   Signs: Unilateral, blood completely fills the clear space between the cornea and conjunctiva.

5. **Dry eye**
   Symptoms: Foreign body sensation, gritty and burning sensation.
   Signs: Bilateral condition, reduced TBUT (<10 seconds), Fl tear prism height is less than 0.2mm at the inferior lid margin, lid wiper epitheliopathy, mucus strands and tear film debris.

2.7 SEVERE PAINFUL RED EYE

1. **Uveitis**
   Symptoms: headache and photophobia.
   Signs: Intraocular inflammation (depending on the area affected), pupillary changes, cells and flare. This condition is subdivided into multiple categories.
   Anterior Uveitis is given as an example below.

   <u>Acute Anterior Uveitis</u>
   Symptoms: Photophobia, dull aching pain (worse when reading/ accommodating), teary eyes and episodes of ocular discomfort a few days before the acute attack.
   Signs: Variable VA (poor VA when there is severe hypopyon), miotic or sluggish pupil, circumcorneal injection, cells and flare in the anterior chamber, posterior synechiae, keratic precipitates and iris nodules (Koeppe/ Busacca).

2. **Anterior Scleritis**
   Subdivided into Non-necrotizing and Necrotizing with inflammation.
   Symptoms: Deep pain (orbit, eyebrow, jaw, temple), tenderness of the globe, photophobia and watery eyes (lacrimation).
   Signs: A gradual VA loss, injection of scleral, episcleral and conjunctival vessels.

   <u>Anterior Non-necrotizing Scleritis</u>
   Usually unilateral, either diffuse or nodular in appearance (scleral nodules do not move over the underlying tissue).
   Diffuse
   Symptoms: Ocular discomfort progressing to aches and pains to the temple and face (worse in the morning but can improve throughout the day).
   Signs: Generalised redness or local to one quadrant.
   Nodular
   Symptoms: A gradual onset of pain, redness and tenderness of the globe.
   Signs: Scleral nodules that are bluish-red and immobile.

   <u>Anterior Necrotizing with Inflammation</u>
   Usually bilateral, pain can be minimal, but VA loss is severe (poor prognosis of recovery).
   Symptoms: A gradual increase in pain, which can extend to the brow, jaw and temple.
   Signs: This can vary depending on the cause; however, the sclera is affected in all cases.

3. **Trauma:** Blunt, Sharp or Chemical Trauma.

   <u>Blunt and Sharp Trauma</u>
   Cause: Squash balls, champagne corks, glass etc.
   Damage depends on which area has been affected and how far it has penetrated the eye.
   Signs: Increased intraocular pressure, corneal abrasion, corneal oedema etc.
   <u>Chemical Trauma</u>
   Injury is related to the property of the chemical itself.
   Symptoms and signs depend on the area affected, how far it has penetrated the eye and the duration of exposure. The outcome can be trivial to potentially blinding.

4. **Contact Lens Related Infiltrate**
   Symptoms: Reduced vision, teary eyes (lacrimation) and photophobia. In some cases, the patient is asymptomatic.
   Signs: Infiltrates are usually observed in the periphery (if central < 2mm in size), conjunctival hyperaemia and discharge observed. (Key point: No anterior cells will be present.)

5. **Corneal Ulcer**
   Symptoms: Photophobia and teary eyes (lacrimation).
   Signs: Ulcer (large if >2mm), grey or white, dot-like appearance but can vary depending on the cause, epithelium and/or stromal stain with fluorescein (fuzzy edges), conjunctival redness, may have lid swelling, ptosis, discharge, anterior chamber activity (cells and flare) and a reduction in the visual acuity (if the ulcer is close to the visual axis).

6. **Keratitis**
   Multiple aetiology, photophobia reported and ulcer/ infiltrate observed (shape and size vary). Common examples of Microbial Keratitis are below:

   Bacterial Keratitis
   Symptoms: Photophobia, blurred vision with purulent or mucopurulent discharge.
   Signs: Variable signs depending on the severity and cause of the condition.
   Ranges from infiltrates causing an epithelial defect, stromal oedema and eyelid swelling to scarring, ulceration and secondary conditions such as Anterior Uveitis, Endophthalmitis etc.

   Herpes Simplex Keratitis
   Symptoms: Variable symptoms include pain (burning, irritation), lacrimation, sudden decrease in vision and/or reports of a recurrent cold sore (Optometrist may see a cold sore on examination).
   Signs: Dendritic ulcer/s, keratic precipitates, secondary conditions such as Uveitis, and reduced contrast sensitivity. If not treated, this can lead to a geographic/ amoebic ulcer.

   Herpes Zoster ophthalmicus
   Symptoms: Reduced vision, discomfort and teary eyes (lacrimation).
   Signs: Variable with different severities. Hutchinson's sign (a lesion on the tip of the nose). Keratitis amongst many other secondary conditions seen on examination.

   Protozoa: Acanthamoeba Keratitis
   May have mild signs, but symptoms are severe.
   Symptoms: Usually unilateral, sudden decrease in vision with moderate to severe eye pain (reports difficulty opening eyes), photophobia, no relief in symptoms even after contact lens removal. The patient may report poor lens hygiene, recent corneal trauma or water exposure (swims/ showers with contact lenses and cleans lenses/ case with tap water).
   Signs: Large ulcer with reduced VA (at least a two line reduction in the Snellen chart). This condition can be difficult to diagnose. In the initial stages, the signs are mild and may resemble Viral Conjunctivitis, and then appear like Herpes Simplex Keratitis. If still not managed accordingly, it can progress to stromal penetration with anterior chamber activity (cells, flare and hypopyon).

7. **Closed Angle Glaucoma**
   Symptoms: Halos around lights, transient blurred vision (can be reported as 'misty vision'), ipsilateral frontal headache, ache around the eye and nausea.
   Signs: Fixed mid-dilated pupil (oval and unresponsive to light), raised IOP (>40mmHg), narrow/ closed anterior chamber angles, hypermetropia (positive shift in Rx), circumlimbal injection, corneal oedema, anterior cells and flare, normal disc or disc oedema with venous congestion and haemorrhages.

Important Gems: Recommended Tests
Red Eye: Thorough case history, visual acuity assessment, pupil assessment, intraocular pressure measurements and tear film assessment (FL and lid eversion). Using the Slit lamp, examine the lids, lashes, meibomian glands, conjunctiva, cornea, sclera and anterior chamber (cells and flare).

2.8 OPTIC DISC OEDEMA

Distinguishing features: Swollen disc margin (cannot distinguish margin from the background and disc from the cup), lack of cupping, haemorrhages at the optic nerve head and an enlarged blind spot.

1. **Raised Intracranial Pressure**
    Symptoms: Constant headache, transient loss of vision (lasting a few seconds), sudden onset of diplopia, feeling sleepy, unwell, vomiting (often projectile) and a throbbing sensation often described as a 'whooshing sound'. The headache exacerbates in the morning, with head movements, coughing or straining.
    Signs: Usually bilateral, asymmetrical, pupillary changes, and an enlarged blind spot. Fundus examination reveals papilloedema consisting of severe disc hyperaemia, blurred disc margins and disc elevation without a physiological cup.
2. **Acute Closed Angle Glaucoma**
    Symptoms: Halos around lights, transient blurred vision (can be reported as 'misty vision'), ipsilateral frontal headache, severe eye pain (ache around the eye) and nausea.
    Signs: Fixed mid-dilated pupil (oval and unresponsive to light), raised IOP (>40mmHg), narrow/ closed anterior chamber angles, hypermetropia (positive shift in Rx), circumlimbal injection, corneal oedema, anterior cells and flare, normal disc or disc oedema with venous congestion and haemorrhages.
3. **Malignant Hypertensive Retinopathy**
    Symptoms: Severe headache, variable loss of vision, nausea and vomiting.
    Signs: Macula star, disc oedema, arterial narrowing, haemorrhages, CWS and exudates. Signs of Non-Malignant HR will also be present e.g. arteriolar tortuosity, arteriosclerosis.
4. **Occlusion**

CRAO
   Symptoms: Sudden, painless, unilateral loss of vision. A ring of blindness that progresses inwards from the periphery towards the centre, can take two hours to progress or notice upon waking. This can be seen as a complete/ transient loss of vision or vision that resolves spontaneously.
   Signs: Reduced visual acuity (6/60 or less), RAPD in the affected eye, cherry red spot at the macula, the fundus is cloudy or yellow, arteries are the same colour and thickness as veins.

BRAO
   Symptoms: Loss of vision or asymptomatic depending on how peripheral the occlusion is.
   Signs: Reduced visual acuity (if the macula is involved), altitudinal or sectoral visual field loss, yellowing of the affected area of the fundus, sectoral optic atrophy, visible collateral shunt vessels and lipid sheathing of the affected area.

CRVO
   Subdivided into Ischaemic and Non-ischaemic Central Retinal Vein Occlusions
1. **Non-ischaemic CRVO**
   Symptoms: Normal or unilateral blurred vision.
   Signs: Variable VA (ranges from 6/6-CF), RAPD is mild/ absent, retinal oedema, cotton wool spots, haemorrhage (superficial, deep blot or flame-shaped), IRMA, dilated or tortuous veins.
2. **Ischaemic CRVO**
   Symptoms: Sudden and severe reduction in vision often noticed upon waking.
   Signs: Reduced visual acuity (CF or worse), marked RAPD, macula oedema, cotton wool spots, haemorrhage (superficial, deep blot or flame-shaped), IRMA, dilated or tortuous veins.

These signs may obscure the fundus view and are present in all four quadrants.

5. **Posterior Scleritis**
    Symptoms: Severe reduction in vision, painful restriction of eye movements, and diplopia. Signs: Ptosis, proptosis, disc oedema with or without cotton wool spots, macula oedema, exudative retinal detachment, and choroidal folds. Signs and symptoms of Anterior Scleritis can be observed too. In some cases, the patient may present with no obvious abnormalities, e.g. serious symptoms but quiet white eyes.
6. **Optic Neuropathy**
    Subdivided into Arteritic and Non-arteritic Ischaemic Optic Neuropathy

---

Giant Cell Arteritis associated AION
   Symptoms: Headache (frontal/ temporal/ occipital/ generalised) exacerbates when lying down, jaw pain or pain whilst chewing, periocular pain, scalp tenderness and the patient may feel unwell.
   Signs: Sudden severe VA loss, RAPD, swollen 'chalky white' discs with splinter or flame-shaped haemorrhages. For further details, refer to 'Chapter 3, Optic Neuropathy VS Optic Neuritis'.

Non-arteritic Ischaemic Optic Neuropathy (NAION)
   Symptoms: Sudden, painless decrease of vision in the affected eye (within hours to days of initial onset or sudden decrease upon waking) and dyschromatopsia.
   Signs: Disc oedema, with or without splinter haemorrhages and an altitudinal visual field defect (commonly an inferior defect causing an absolute scotoma, but can also be a central, paracentral or arcuate defect).

---

7. **Optic Neuritis**
    Symptoms: Pain with eye movement in extreme gazes, eye and brow pain, headache, blurred vision, impaired night vision, red desaturation (colour appears washed out), and impaired depth perception (difficult to judge distances when walking up and down stairs etc.)
    Signs: Central VA and visual field loss, RAPD if unilateral and a reduction in contrast sensitivity.
8. **Pseudo-papilloedema such as Optic Disc Drusen**
    Symptoms: Often bilateral, asymptomatic with a gradual reduction in the visual field.
    Signs: Swollen (lumpy-bumpy) discs mimic papilloedema (elevated discs with no physiological cup and absent hyperaemia).

This list is not exhaustive.

Important Gems: Recommended Tests
Disc abnormalities
1. Colour vision test: Washed-out image when abnormal.
2. Visual Field tests: Enlarged blind spot when abnormal.
3. Pupil assessment: Relative afferent pupil defect observed.
4. Dilated fundus examination: Always check anterior chamber angles (with Van Herricks) and intraocular pressure before using mydriatic drops.

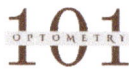

2.9 ABNORMAL PUPILS

1. **Acute Closed Angle Glaucoma**
   Symptoms: Halos around lights, transient blurred vision (can be reported as 'misty vision'), ipsilateral frontal headache, severe eye pain (ache around the eye) and nausea.
   Signs: Fixed mid-dilated pupil (oval and unresponsive to light), raised IOP (>40mmHg), narrow/ closed anterior chamber angles, hypermetropia (positive shift in Rx), circumlimbal injection, corneal oedema, anterior cells and flare, normal disc or disc oedema with venous congestion and haemorrhages.
2. **Raised Intracranial Pressure**
   Symptoms: Constant headache, transient loss of vision (lasting a few seconds), sudden onset of diplopia, feeling sleepy, unwell, vomiting (often projectile) and a throbbing sensation often described as a 'whooshing sound'. The headache exacerbates in the morning, with head movements, coughing or straining.
   Signs: Usually bilateral, asymmetrical, with an enlarged blind spot. Fundus examination reveals papilloedema consisting of severe disc hyperaemia, blurred disc margins and disc elevation without a physiological cup.
3. **Uveitis**
   Symptoms: Headache, pain, a red eye and photophobia.
   Signs: Intraocular inflammation (depending on the area affected), cells and flare. This condition is subdivided into multiple categories. Anterior Uveitis is given as an example below. For further details, refer to 'Chapter 3, Uveitis'.

> **Acute Anterior Uveitis**
> **Symptoms**: Photophobia, dull aching pain (worse when reading/ accommodating), a red eye, teary eyes (lacrimation) and episodes of ocular discomfort a few days before the acute attack.
> **Signs**: Variable VA (poor VA when there is severe hypopyon), miotic or sluggish pupil, circumcorneal injection, cells and flare in the anterior chamber, posterior synechiae, keratic precipitates, and iris nodules (Koeppe/ Busacca).

4. **Third Nerve Palsy**
   Symptoms: Sudden onset of diplopia, reports of tilting the head to either reduce diplopia or separate the double image so that it is easier to distinguish them.
   Signs: EOM affected (SR, MR, IR, IO). The affected eye is **down and out,** with ptosis, mydriasis, paresis of accommodation and loss of pupil action (fixed, dilated pupils).
5. **Adie Pupil**
   Symptoms: Photophobia, blurred vision and difficulty adapting to the dark.
   Signs: Usually unilateral, the affected pupil is larger than normal with an absent or sluggish response to light but preserved near response.
6. **Horner's Syndrome**
   Signs: Usually unilateral, miosis of the affected eye (more evident in dim light as the Horner pupil cannot dilate) with normal pupillary reactions to light and near. Irides are different in colour (the affected eye is lighter), mild ptosis and mild elevation of the inferior eyelid.
7. **Argyll Robertson Pupils**
   Signs: Bilateral miosis with little or no constriction to direct light. In dim light, pupils remain small and can be irregular.
8. **Conditions affecting the optic nerve**
   Certain infections, inflammatory diseases, tumours etc.

Important Gems: Recommended Tests
Abnormal Pupils: Visual field test, colour vision test, pupil assessment, dilated fundus examination and anterior chamber assessment.

RAPD

1. **Retinal Detachment**
   Subdivided into Rhegmatogenous, Tractional and Exudative Retinal Detachment.
   Symptoms: Flashes (photopsia), floaters, shadows or 'curtain in their vision'.
   Signs: Sudden decrease in VA and visual field (if the macula is involved), tobacco dust, lower IOP in the affected eye (can be 5mmHg lower), a RAPD can occur when the macula or two quadrants of the retina are detached, retinal tears, breaks or holes, macula on/ off and may have vitreoretinal degeneration (lattice degeneration etc.)
2. **Occlusion:** Arterial occlusions (CRAO/ BRAO) and Ischaemic Vein Occlusions.

CRAO
Symptoms: Sudden, painless, unilateral loss of vision. A ring of blindness that progresses inwards from the periphery towards the centre, can take two hours to progress or notice upon waking, seen as a complete/ transient loss of vision or vision that resolves spontaneously.
Signs: VA loss (6/60 or less), RAPD in the affected eye, swollen disc, cherry red spot at the macula, the fundus is cloudy or yellow, arteries are the same colour and thickness as veins.

BRAO
Symptoms: Loss of vision or asymptomatic depending on how peripheral the occlusion is.
Signs: Reduced Visual acuity (if the macula is involved), altitudinal or sectoral visual field loss, yellowing of the affected area of the fundus, sectoral optic atrophy, visible collateral shunt vessels and lipid sheathing of the affected area.

CRVO: Subdivided into Ischaemic and Non-ischaemic Central Retinal Vein Occlusion.
- **Non-ischaemic CRVO**
  Symptoms: Normal or unilateral blurred vision.
  Signs: Variable VA (6/6-CF), RAPD (mild/ absent), retinal and disc oedema (mild/ absent), CWS, haemorrhages (superficial, deep blot, flame-shaped), IRMA, dilated or tortuous veins.
- **Ischaemic CRVO**
  Symptoms: Sudden and severe reduction in vision often noticed upon waking.
  Signs: Reduced VA (CF or worse), RAPD, wavy lines on Amsler, severe disc and macula oedema, CWS, haemorrhages (superficial, deep blot or flame-shaped), IRMA, dilated and tortuous veins.   These signs may obscure the fundus view and are present in all 4 quadrants.

3. **End-stage Glaucoma**
   Symptoms: Variable, ranging from tunnel vision (permanent loss of vision) to difficulty adapting to low light. Patient's lifestyle will be debilitated (symptoms will represent this).
   Signs: VA and VF severely reduced and permanent optic nerve head damage. In some cases, a RAPD is observed, e.g. during a substantial progression of Primary Open Angle Glaucoma.
4. **Severe Macular Degeneration**
   Symptoms: Central scotoma, visual distortions and difficulty adapting to low light levels.
   Signs: RAPD (if unilateral and severe) with poor VA. (Other signs of MD present too).
5. **Giant Cell Arteritis associated AION**
   Symptoms: Headache (frontal/ temporal/ occipital/ generalised) exacerbates when lying down, jaw pain or pain whilst chewing, periocular pain and scalp tenderness.
   Signs: Sudden severe VA loss, swollen 'chalky white' discs with splinter or flame-shaped haemorrhages. For further details, refer to 'Chapter 3, Optic Neuropathy VS Optic Neuritis'.
6. **Optic Neuritis**
   Symptoms: Pain with eye movement in extreme gazes, eye and brow pain, headache, blurred vision, impaired night vision, red desaturation (colour appears washed out), and impaired depth perception (difficult to judge distances when walking up and down stairs etc.)
   Signs: Central vision and visual field loss, reduction in contrast sensitivity, RAPD if unilateral and optic nerve swelling (Papillitis or Neuroretinitis).

2.10 IS THE LESION CANCEROUS?

Non-cancerous

Chalazion (Meibomian Cyst)
Symptoms: Slow-growing eyelid nodule/s, variable pain (eyelid discomfort, irritation, teary eyes or painless). May report previous occurrences of eyelid swelling/ nodules.
Signs: Non-tender eyelid nodule in the tarsal plate, commonly affecting the upper lid.
Large Chalazia: Can cause astigmatism, hyperopia, and blurred vision. This is due to the nodule pressing against the eyeball, distorting the cornea.
Advice: This is a recurrent condition, to be aware if similar signs and symptoms occur.
Management
- ❖ If small and asymptomatic: Self-limiting (within weeks to months).
  Hygiene measures are necessary to prevent reoccurrences. Always keep the area clean and avoid touching the eyes/ using contaminated eye cosmetics etc.
- ❖ Symptomatic relief: Lid massages, warm compresses or steroid eye drops/ ointments.
- ❖ For recurrent, large, or non-resolving chalazia: Refer to HES.

RPE Hypertrophy
Subdivided into Typical and Atypical Hypertrophy.
This is a tumour of the retinal pigment epithelium/ benign lesion/s.
Signs: Flat, dark grey or black, round or oval with defined margins and roughly 1–3 disc diameter in size.

Choroidal Naevus
Usually seen at birth, this can increase in size during pre-pubertal years; however, growth is minimal by adulthood. If there is an increase in size in adulthood, refer to the HES to rule out melanoma.
Symptoms: Usually asymptomatic, however picked up during the routine sight test.
Signs: Brown to slate grey, 2-5 disc diameter in size, oval or circular, indistinct margins, flat or slightly elevated, and surface drusen may be visible too.

Management: Routine referral to confirm the diagnosis and monitor regularly (visual field assessment, fundus examination, OCT). Always record size, colour and location.

Cancerous/ Malignant Tumours

Choroidal Melanoma
Symptoms: Reduced vision, metamorphopsia, visual field loss, flashes (photopsia) and floaters. In some cases, the patient is asymptomatic.
Signs: White or greenish grey, >10 disc diameter in size, significantly elevated, pigmented, may have overlying Serous Detachment, Secondary Glaucoma, Rubeosis iridis, Cataract, intraocular inflammation etc.

Basal Cell Carcinoma
Symptoms: usually asymptomatic.
Signs: Slow developing, non-resolving lesion of the eyelid skin.
- ❖ **Nodular:** hard nodule with a pearly appearance.
- ❖ **Nodulo- ulcerative**: Nodular but with a raised central ulcer which may bleed.
- ❖ **Morphoeic/ sclerosing**: Flat and hardened plaque of thickened skin.

Advise: Sun protection measures and reassure the patient that this is low-risk skin cancer.

Management: Refer with details of location, size, previous history and observations.

HOW TO DIFFERENTIATE...

3.1 CATARACT
The three most common forms seen in practice are described below:

Cortical Cataract
Risk factors
- Age, female, and family history of the condition.

Symptoms
- Glare whilst driving at night and difficulty reading (worse in dim light).
- Monocular diplopia (usually in the early stages of the condition).

Signs
- Wedge-shaped or radial spoke-like opacities in the periphery of the crystalline lens.
- Rx change, astigmatic change and sector visual field loss.
- Contrast sensitivity can be affected.

Management
- Protection from ultraviolet radiation is advised and avoid tinted sunglasses.
- Reduce the interval for the next sight test.

Nuclear Sclerotic Cataract
Risk factors
- Age and smoking.

Symptoms
- Difficulty reading, glare and a reduction in colour vision.

Signs
- Increased yellowing and brunescence of the crystalline lens.
  When advanced, it can appear brown/ black on slit lamp biomicroscopy.
- Rx change, myopic shift (the second sight of the aged) and diffuse visual field loss.
- Red desaturation.

Management
- Advise tints, protection from UV exposure, and reduct the interval for the next sight test.
- Counsel: Methods to increase lighting whilst reading and implications of smoking.

Posterior Subcapsular Cataract
Risk factors
- Age (can occur amongst the working age group).
- Ocular diseases (e.g. RP), Diabetes (causes metabolic cataract/ snowflake cortical opacities).
- Side effects of steroid use, e.g. longterm use of oral corticosteroids can cause a toxic cataract.
- Lifestyle factors, e.g. smoking.

Symptoms
- Difficulty reading, glare particularly under conditions of miosis, i.e. bright sunlight.

Signs
- Vacuolated, granular-like appearance on slit lamp biomicroscopy.
- Dramatic reduction in VA (NV>DV), diffuse VF loss and a reduction in contrast sensitivity.

Management
- Write to the GP if a PSC cataract is associated with steroid use.
- Advice: Tints and protection from ultraviolet radiation is advised. Warn patients about the implications of smoking and reduce the interval for the next sight test.

Important Gems: When to refer for Cataract Surgery?
- When the desired lifestyle is debilitated.
- When vision is impaired (VA 6/9 or worse) or there is a reduction in contrast sensitivity affecting the patient's quality of life.
- When there is a dense or mature cataract (the crystalline lens is completely opaque).
- When BV is affected, i.e. with a unilateral cataract, be mindful that an exotropia can develop.

The Benefits of Referring for Cataract Surgery!
- The First Eye: Improves visual acuity and reduces glare.
- The Second Eye: Binocular consideration (the patient maintains stereopsis), prevents anisometropia, disabling glare and improves contrast sensitivity.
- Always refer for treatment to remove the opacity at the earliest opportunity.
  Avoid prescribing spectacles when a referral is being made.
  Always include in the referral letter that the patient would like to be considered for surgery.
  Usually, refer for one eye first, but you can refer for both eyes if they both meet the standard.

ADDITIONAL NOTES

3.2 GLAUCOMA

Normal IOP
- The average IOP is between 15-16mmHg but this can range between 10-21mmHg.
- A difference in IOP between the two eyes (<4 mmHg).
- IOP can be reduced by exercise & accommodation and increased by drinking & lying down.
- Always consider corneal thickness alongside IOP.
  (Thinner corneas underestimate IOP, and thicker corneas overestimate IOP)

Normal NRR examination: Always use the other eye as a reference for comparison.
- The average horizontal/vertical CD ratio is 0.3-0.4. The horizontal CD ratio is generally larger (less than 5% of normal patients have a CD ratio >0.65).
- Asymmetry in the CD ratio of <0.2 between the two eyes.
- ISNT rule followed: (inferior ≥ superior ≥ nasal ≥ temporal).
- Normal variations of an optic cup: Dimple with a small central cup, punched out with a larger or deeper cup or a sloping temporal wall.
- Peripapillary changes: Examine the edge of the ONH (alpha is darker than beta PPA).

Primary Open Angle Glaucoma

Risk factors
- Afro-Caribbean: Disease starts at a younger age (approximately ten years earlier than other ethnicities), with higher presenting IOPs, more severe disc changes, thinner corneas, more resistance to treatment and a worse prognosis.
- FH: First-degree relatives are at an increased risk (parent, sibling or child with Glaucoma).
- Myopia and age (increased risk after 60+).
- Low CCT underestimates IOP, causing a higher glaucoma risk if it remains undiagnosed.
- Secondary factors: Diabetes, vascular diseases, hypothyroidism, Raynauds Syndrome.

Symptoms
No/ minimal symptoms reported until the disease has advanced, then there are reports of tunnel vision etc.

Signs
1. **Glaucomatous Optic Nerve Damage**
   - Greater the CD ratio, the higher the risk (>0.6), vertical elongation of the cup (oval).
   - Cupping: Consider size of disc (large/ moderate/ small) alongside damage of the NRR.
   - Asymmetry in the CD Ratio: >0.2 between the two eyes.
   - ISNT rule <u>NOT</u> followed: Thinning of NRR, damage commonly occurs inferiorly and superiorly first, as well as notching, which produces a wedge-shaped (arcuate) defect.
2. **Lamina cribrosa and PPA** (Beta PPA is more glaucomatous, white/ light in appearance)
3. **Vascular clinical changes**
   - A nasal shift of disc vessels.
   - Baring: Enlarged cup leaving vessels hanging mid-air (early glaucomatous sign).
   - Bayonetting: The vessel has a 'z' appearance at the edge of the cup.
   - Splinter haemorrhage: Flame-shaped, location (IT/ST) and commonly seen in NTG.
4. **Visual field loss corresponding to optic nerve damage**: Paracentral scotoma, arcuate scotoma, nasal step, a ring scotoma (advanced stage) etc.
5. **Raised IOP:** >24mmHg
6. **Anterior chamber:** Open anterior chamber angle (grade 4 in Van Herricks).

Refer
- IOP > 30, irrespective of other risks.
- IOP > 24 if there are other risks too.
- Any IOP if there is evidence of optic nerve damage or there is a difference of >4mmHg between the two eyes.

Primary Angle Closure Glaucoma

Subdivided into Acute (AACG), Intermittent (IACG) and Chronic (CACG).
This condition is caused by an IOP increase due to an obstruction of aqueous outflow by partial or complete closure of the angle by the peripheral iris.

Risk factors
- Female, asain ethnicity and hypermetropia.
- FH: First-degree relatives are at an increased risk (parent, sibling or child with Glaucoma).
- Shallow anterior chamber: With age, the AC becomes shallower as lens thickness increases.
- Use of sympathomimetics.

Stages
1. **Prodromal**
   The reported symptoms are vague, e.g. ocular discomfort and intermittent headache.
   However, in many cases, patients are asymptomatic.
   Sign: Narrow anterior chamber angles (capable of closure).
2. **Sub-acute**
   Episodes of haloes around lights (rainbow-coloured rings around white light),
   misty vision lasting 1-2 hours, ache in the eye and a temporal headache.
   (These symptoms may occur when the pupil dilates, i.e. in low lighting)
3. **Acute attack**

Sx   Halos around lights, a sudden decrease or transient loss of blurred vision,
intense eye pain (ocular, periocular), ipsilateral frontal headache, nausea and vomiting.
The patient reports a history of previous intermittent (sub-acute) attacks.

Signs
- Hypermetropia (positive shift in Rx) and reduced visual acuity (6/60 to HM).
- Mid-dilated fixed pupils (vertically oval and unresponsive to light).
- Narrow/ closed angle in the anterior chamber (Grade 0/ 1/ 2 in Van Herricks).
- Circumlimbal redness, ciliary flush, corneal oedema, anterior cells and flare.
- Fundus: Normal discs or disc oedema with venous congestion & haemorrhages.
- Raised IOP: >40 mmHg.

4. **Post attack:** Poor VA, a non-reactive or sluggish pupil with or without iris atrophy.

Management
- This depends on the type of attack and if previously seen at the hospital eye service (HES).
- Acute attack warrants first aid and emergency referral to the HES.

Ocular Hypertension
Raised intraocular pressure (IOP) with no clinical optic nerve head damage or visual field defect.
- Refer if IOP > 24 mmHg (aim to repeat with Goldman and refer on repeated IOP).
- Approximately 10% of ocular hypertensives will develop Glaucoma in five years.

Normal Tension Glaucoma
Intraocular pressure (IOP) is within normal limits, and open anterior chamber angles; however, the optic nerve will show damage and signs of Glaucoma.
- A common sign is splinter haemorrhages at the disc (location commonly IT/ ST).
- These patients typically have a thicker central corneal thickness.
- Early visual field defect: superonasally (paracentral defect).

Pseudo-exfoliation Glaucoma
Dandruff-like material on the pupil margin or anterior lens capsule.
- IOP > 21 mmHg, mild flare and narrow anterior chamber angles.
- Optic nerve head damage and visual field loss similar to Primary Open Angle Glaucoma.

Important Gems: Secondary Glaucoma
Secondary Glaucoma may present similar signs and symptoms as explained in 'Chapter 3, Glaucoma'. Always remain vigilant and remember that conditions can coincide or occur in isolation. Full history from the patient is vital to eliminate/ diagnose the origin of conditions, e.g. a patient using long-term steroids can get Secondary Glaucoma.

Relevant tests: IOP (Goldman), visual field assessment (refer when there are repeatable visual field defects), optic nerve assessment (dilated examination) and assessment of the anterior chamber angle.

ADDITIONAL NOTES

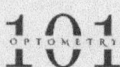

3.3 DIABETIC RETINOPATHY

Risk factors
- Diabetes (duration and poor control increases the risk of Diabetic Retinopathy).
- Hypertension, anaemia, pregnancy and lifestyle factors, e.g. smoking, obesity.

1. **Background Diabetic Retinopathy: Minimal or Mild Non-proliferative BDR**
   Symptoms: Usually asymptomatic.
   Signs are subdivided into:
   Minimal BDR
   - Microaneurysms only (small, red dot-like appearance which is remarkably similar in appearance to dot haemorrhages).

   Mild non-proliferative BDR: Microaneurysms and one or more of:
   - Hard exudates: Yellow/ white spots, waxy lesions with distinct edges, defined margins, in clumps together or as rings often surrounded by microaneurysms.
   - Cotton wool spots: White fluffy, superficial lesions with indistinct margins that can obscure underlying blood vessels, larger and more spread out compared to drusen.
   - Dot/ small blot haemorrhages: bigger than dot haemorrhages with indistinct margins.
   - Flame-shaped haemorrhages
   - Intraretinal haemorrhages

2. **Pre-Proliferative Diabetic Retinopathy**
   Greater number of signs (in all quadrants) of mild non-proliferative BDR as well as:
   - Intraretinal microvascular abnormalities (IRMA): Resembles new vessel growth but does not cross over major retinal blood vessels. Red, irregular, line-like appearance found between arterioles and venues.
   - Venous changes, e.g. dilation, beading and looping.
   - Arterial changes, e.g. narrowing of blood vessels.
   - Dark blot and dot haemorrhages.

3. **Proliferative Diabetic Retinopathy**
   Symptoms: Blurred and/ or fluctuating vision reported.
   Signs: neovascularisation.
   - NVD: New vessels on the disc or within 1 disc diameter (DD) of the disc.
     (Total area equates to approximately **1/3DD in size**).
   - NVE: New vessels along the course of major vessels.
     (Total area equates to approximately **1/2DD in size**).
   - Other secondary causes of proliferative DR, e.g. Uveitis, Cataract surgery and vein occlusions. Pre-proliferative and Background Diabetic Retinopathy signs will be visible in all four quadrants. *All these signs occur away from the macula.*

4. **Advanced Proliferative Diabetic Retinopathy**
   - NVD > 1/3DD in size or NVE > 1/2DD in size.
   - Any NVD or NVE (>1/2DD in size) with pre-retinal or vitreous haemorrhage.
   - Rubeosis iridis: New vessels on the iris. This can progress to Neovascular Glaucoma.
   - Fibrosis: Less likely to bleed but more likely to lead to Tractional Retinal Detachment.

Referral Guidelines
- **Routine referral:** Background Diabetic Retinopathy.
- **Referral within four weeks:** Unexplained drop in vision, hard exudates within 1DD of the fovea, macula oedema, pre-proliferative or severe DR, and unexplained retinal findings.
- **Referral within one week:** Proliferative signs of Diabetic Retinopathy.

3.4 DIABETIC MACULOPATHY

This is based on Retinopathy seen at the macula and can cause visual impairment in diabetic patients.

Different types of Diabetic Maculopathy
1. **Focal**: Hard exudates (rings or incomplete rings) and macula oedema within one disc diameter (DD) of the fovea.
2. **Ischaemic**: Reduced vision, microaneurysms, cotton wool spots and IRMA.
3. **Cystoid**: Microaneurysms, dot or blot haemorrhages **and** reduced VA (6/12 or worse).
4. **Diffused**: Generalised oedema, haemorrhages and any of the signs above.

Clinically Significant Signs
- Any microaneurysm/ haemorrhage within 1DD of the macula **with** a VA less than 6/12.
- Any exudates within 1DD of the centre of the fovea.
- A group of exudates within the area of the macula.
    (If there are exudates outside of these areas and no other signs, then it is not clinically significant macular oedema).

Relevant Tests
1. **Visual Acuity Testing**
   A patient with Maculopathy will have reduced central vision and difficulty seeing fine details, e.g. recognising faces and reading small prints.
2. **Contrast Sensitivity Tests**
   These tests are sensitive indicators of early macular dysfunction. Suppose a patient has good visual acuity (6/6 recorded on the Snellen chart) but low contrast sensitivity, this explains the symptoms of poor vision reported by the patient.
3. **Fundus Biomicroscopy (VOLK):** Use a red-free filter to examine the fundus more clearly.
4. **Other tests:** Amsler test and colour vision tests.

Effects of Diabetes
- Refractive changes: Transient myopic shift in Rx with increasing hyperglycaemia.
  A patient whose blood sugar levels are not controlled during the eye examination will give a variable refraction. For this reason, refer to the GP first to control blood sugar levels, then repeat refraction once the levels are controlled before issuing new glasses.
- Corneal changes, e.g. decrease in sensitivity.
- Cataract: Age-related Cataract occurs earlier in diabetic patients. They are also more prone to nuclear lens opacities. A classical Diabetic Cataract is a snowflake Cataract which may mature within a few days but can resolve spontaneously.
- Glaucoma: There is a two-three times greater risk of Primary Open Angle Glaucoma for diabetic patients. Rubeosis iridis or new vessels in the angle of the anterior chamber can cause Secondary Angle Closure Glaucoma.
- Cranial Nerve Palsy: Can cause pupil-sparing Third Nerve Palsy.

Difference between Diabetic Retinopathy and Hypertensive Retinopathy
1. **Diabetic Retinopathy presents with a 'wet' retina.**
   Observe multiple haemorrhages, multiple exudates, extensive oedema, and a few cotton wool spots. These patients rarely present with flame-shaped haemorrhages (unless there is co-existing Hypertensive Retinopathy) and abnormal retinal veins and capillaries.
2. **Hypertensive Retinopathy presents with a 'dry' retina.**
   Observe a few haemorrhages, oedema is rare, exudates are rare, and multiple cotton wool spots. These patients also present with flame-shaped haemorrhages and abnormalities of the retinal arteries. Hypertensive Retinopathy is a bilateral, very symmetrical condition.

3.5 HYPERTENSIVE RETINOPATHY

Subdivided into Non-malignant and Malignant Hypertensive Retinopathy
Risk factors
- Afro-Caribbean, raised blood pressure (BP) and family history of the condition.
- Lifestyle factors, e.g. smoking, obesity, alcohol.

Non-malignant Hypertensive Retinopathy
Signs
1. **Arteriolar narrowing**: Generalised (grade I) or focal (grade II).
   - Salus sign: Pressure leading to deflection of the vein from its normal path.
   - Gunn sign: Localised narrowing of the vein as it passes under the arteriole.
   - Bonnet sign: Collection of blood from the vein beyond the crossing (i.e. further away from the optic disc), causing the distal part of the vein to be thicker than the proximal part.
2. **Arteriosclerosis**
   Width of the arterial reflex as a ratio of the arterial calibre (20-30% is normal).
3. **Arteriolar tortuosity**: 0 (no tortuosity) to 4 (severe tortuosity), segmental or uniform throughout the retina (segmental arteriolar tortuosity is commonly seen in the nasal retina).

(Always describe the severity using a 5-point grading scale)

Malignant Hypertensive Retinopathy (Grade III)
Sx   Severe headaches, variable vision loss, nausea and vomiting.
Signs
Grade II as well as:
- Arterial narrowing and arteriovenous nipping: Copper wiring (A:V ratio of 25%), silver wiring and/ or distal banking.
- Cotton wool spots, hard exudates and haemorrhages (dot, blot and flame-shaped).
- In rare cases, there can be retinal and macular oedema.

(Record the presence of these lesions along with their number, size, and location).

Advanced Malignant Hypertensive Retinopathy (Grade IV)
Signs
- Disc oedema
- Macular star: Ring of exudates from the disc to the macula.

Management
Refer to the cardiologist to rule out ischaemia and refer to the GP to treat or diagnose any underlying hypertension.
- Non-urgent basis: Grade I/ II
- Urgent referral to the GP: Grade III
- Medical crisis to the hospital eye service (HES): Grade IV (involving disc oedema)

Prognosis: Changes following blood pressure (BP) control through treatment.
- Swollen disc   Develops within days to weeks of elevated BP and resolves within months following BP lowering.
- Macula star   Appear within several weeks of elevated BP and resolves within months to years following BP lowering.
- Exudates   Even after treatment, these hard exudates can last over 12 months.
- CWS   Appear within 1-2 days of elevated BP and resolves within 2-10 weeks following BP lowering.

RPE disruption at the macula or optic nerve damage can limit visual recovery.

Important Gems: How to measure the A:V ratio (width of an artery to vein).
Compare adjacent arteries and veins and the equivalent number of bifurcations of the two vessels, 1–3 disc diameters from the optic disc. 100% represents equality, and 50% represents an arterial calibre that is half that of a vein, which indicates the amount of arteriosclerosis.
An A:V ratio of 2:3 is normal.

ADDITIONAL NOTES

3.6 MACULAR DEGENERATION

Subdivided into Dry and Wet Age-related Macular Degeneration (AMD)
Risk factors
- Age (increased risk after 45).
- Caucasian: Higher prevalence of large drusen, pigmentary changes and Wet AMD.
- Family history (increased risk if a first-degree relative has the condition).
- Sunlight exposure
- Female
- Hypertension and high cholesterol.
- Lifestyle factors, e.g. smoking accelerates the development of Wet and Dry forms of AMD.

Dry AMD
Symptoms
- Difficulty recognising faces and reading (positive scotoma). The patient may struggle to adapt to bright light, and there is a gradual change in vision (over months-years).
- In some cases, patients are asymptomatic until the condition becomes advanced.

Signs   Soft drusen ➡ Confluent drusen ➡ RPE Atrophy ➡ Geographic Atrophy (late stages)

1. Drusen: The first clinically detectable sign of AMD.
    - Hard/ small drusen: Discrete whitish-yellow spots, glistening appearance with sharp boundaries.
    - Soft/ large drusen: Indistinct edges, yellow or white, are more confluent and are usually larger than hard drusen. The presence of this drusen can increase the likelihood of the progression to advanced AMD within five years.

    Large numbers of small hard drusen (≥ 8) increase the risk of developing into soft drusen and/ or AMD within fifteen years.
2. RPE degeneration: A variable amount of hyper/ hypopigmentation (sharply demarcated pale areas and pigment clumps) eventually leading to atrophy of the overlying RPE. Choroidal vessels are sometimes visible.
3. Increased accumulation of debris under the retina.
4. Geographic atrophy: Advanced stage of AMD at the retinal pigment epithelium (RPE). If longstanding dark-pigmented margins are visible.
5. Central visual field loss and visual acuity worse than 6/60 (unless there is foveal sparing).

Signs are usually seen in both eyes but are asymmetrical.

Management
Advice: Methods to increase lighting whilst reading, protection from UV radiation in Rx, LVAs, higher reading adds, having a diet containing green leafy vegetables and supplements with lutein and zeaxanthin. Advice about the risk of Wet AMD and implications of smoking.
Counsel: Optometrists cannot give stronger prescription glasses to improve vision, reassuring the patient that the condition will progress slowly and central vision is affected only.
Refer: To confirm the diagnosis, low vision assessment and certification for sight impairment.
Register: With Social Services for financial help, practical mobility training etc.
Monitor: Must self-monitor using an Amsler chart and return immediately if changes occur.

Distinguishing between Exudates and Drusens
Hard exudates
- Intraretinal ring pattern with vascular changes.
- Additional findings: Microaneurysms, cotton wool spots, dot and blot haemorrhages.

Hard drusen
- Sub-retinal random pattern with no vascular changes initially.

Wet AMD

Symptoms
- Sudden onset of distorted monocular vision (straight lines appear wavy or crooked) and positive scotoma (if haemorrhages are present).

Signs
- A hyperopic shift in the Rx.
- Exudated serous and blood (red if subretinal, darker if sub-RPE).
- Cotton wool spots (if ischaemic).
- Raised macula area.
- Choroidal Neo-vascularisation: The membrane can have a green, grey or pinkish-yellow appearance, but often this is difficult to see (easier with fluorescein angiography).
  - **Classic**: Clearly demarcated borders (intensity increases and size remains constant).
  - **Occult**: Poorly demarcated borders, source undetermined, late leakage and elevation of the retinal pigment epithelium.
- Exudative detachment of the retinal pigment epithelium.
- Disciform scar (late stage): Circular shape, defined margins, pale yellow or white, irregular elevated surface, patches or pools of subretinal blood may be visible. This causes permanent loss of vision (CF or HM); at this stage, the patient is unsuitable for treatment.

Management
- The symptoms alone merit an urgent referral, even without any signs.

ADDITIONAL NOTES

3.7 VITREOUS DETACHMENT

Vitreous Opacities

- **Weiss ring**: Imprint of the optic disc attachment on the vitreous gel.
- **Haemorrhage**: retro-vitreal (pre-retinal)/ intra-vitreal.
- **Asteroid hyalosis:** White or yellow, shiny round opacities (size can vary), do not settle at rest and are usually seen in diabetic patients.
- **Synchisis scintillans:** Golden crystals that settle inferiorly with rest and are associated with chronic vitreous haemorrhages.
- **Muscae Volitantes/ floaters:** Thread-like appearance (often described as a cobweb or fly) noticeable when looking at a plain uniformed background. A sudden increase can be caused by a posterior vitreous detachment, haemorrhage, retinal tissue etc.
- **Tobacco dust:** Brown RPE cells and flare (Schaffer's sign) in the anterior vitreous.
    If seen, assume a retinal break is present unless proven otherwise.

Vitreous Degeneration

1. **Syneresis**: Condensation of the vitreous gel.
Cause   Age, myopia and trauma.
Sx   Sudden onset of floaters (dots, circles, lines or shadows in the patient's vision).

2. **Posterior Vitreous detachment:** Occurs with or without vitreous gel collapse.
Cause   Diabetes, age, synchysis (vitreous gel liquefaction), syneresis, myopia,
          post-inflammatory, post-vitreous haemorrhage etc.
Sx   Sudden onset of flashing lights (photopsia) which can be triggered by head/eye movement
          Floaters: Dot/ thread-like appearance (often described as a cobweb or fly) in their vision.
Signs   Weiss ring (large ring/ circle imprint of the optic disc attachment on the vitreous gel).
   PVD <u>WITH</u> Gel Collapse
   - If vitreous haemorrhages are present the patient may report blurred vision, blood and pigments are observed in the anterior vitreous, and 20% develop into a retinal break.
   - If no vitreous haemorrhages are present, 4% develop into a retinal break.

   PVD <u>WITHOUT</u> Gel Collapse
   - Scaffold for proliferative new vessels.
   - Associated with future retinal holes and vitreous haemorrhages.

Vitreous Haemorrhage

Causes
- Proliferative Retinopathies: Diabetes, Retinal Vein Occlusion, Sickle Cell Retinopathy.
- Other causes: PVD, Disciform Macular Degeneration, Blood Dyscrasias and trauma.

Complications
- Syneresis and fibrosis can cause Tractional Retinal Detachment.

Management
1. Follow the emergency referral protocol if there is any suspicion of a tear.
   Undergo the following tests to rule out a Retinal Detachment.
   - Dilated fundoscopy (examine all extreme gaze positions).
   - Tonometry and slit lamp biomicroscopy.
   - Visual field and visual acuity assessment.
2. Review patients with acute onset PVDs one month after the initial onset.
3. Caution the patient to return immediately if symptoms change, e.g. increasing floaters, flashing lights, shadow, or curtain in their vision.

ADDITIONAL NOTES

3.8 RETINAL DETACHMENT

Subdivided into Rhegmatogenous, Tractional and Exudative Retinal Detachment

Rhegmatogenous Retinal Detachment
Following a PVD, fluid from the vitreous enters the subretinal space through a tear or hole. This can cause vitreous haemorrhaging, traction and the collection of subretinal fluid, which causes a Retinal Detachment. To relieve traction, a retinal break, tear or hole forms.
Risk factor
- PVD, myopia, and patients with predisposing lesions, e.g. lattice degeneration.

Symptoms
- Photopsia (flashes), floaters, shadows or 'curtain in their vision'.
  To note: 60% of patients with a Retinal Detachment have ALL these symptoms.

Signs
- A sudden decrease in VA (if the macula is involved) and a relative visual field defect.
- Lower IOP in the affected eye: Approximately 5mmHg lower compared to the other eye.
- Tobacco dust (Schaefer's sign): Brown RPE cells in the anterior vitreous.
- May suffer from mild Anterior Uveitis.
- A RAPD is usually seen when the macula or two quadrants of the retina is detached.
- Fundus examination: Opaque appearance due to oedema, macular on/ off, retinal tears, breaks or holes visible (u-shaped tear, atrophic hole, operculated etc.)
  (Retinal breaks occur soon after the onset of a PVD but can also occur after several weeks).
- May have vitreoretinal degeneration, e.g. lattice degeneration.

Management
- An emergency referral is necessary.
- Include in the referral letter whether the macula is still on/off as a 'Retinal Detachment with macula on' warrants immediate management for a better prognosis in vision.

Complications of surgery: Anterior or posterior segment ischaemia, infections, muscle imbalance, refractive changes, macula pucker, Cataract and Glaucoma.

Tractional Retinal Detachment
The neurosensory retina is pulled away from the RPE and there are no retinal breaks.
Cause   Penetrating ocular trauma, proliferative retinopathies, vitreous haemorrhage etc.
          (not associated with an acute posterior vitreous detachment)

Symptoms
- Progressive visual field loss.   To note: Photopsia and floaters are usually absent.

Signs
- Breaks are usually absent, but signs appear similar to Rhegmatogenous Retinal Detachment if there is a break.

Exudative Retinal Detachment
Subretinal fluid from the neurosensory retinal and choroidal vessels builds up in the subretinal space.
Cause   Choroidal tumours, inflammatory conditions, subretinal neovascularization etc.

Symptoms
- Floaters (if there is Vitritis).   To note: No flashes will be reported.
- A visual field defect can develop suddenly and will progress rapidly.

Signs
- Smooth retinal surface (no folds, breaks or holes).
- This can be bilateral (depending on the cause).
  The cause itself may be seen when examining the eye, e.g. if a choroidal tumour is the cause, this will be observed when undergoing a fundus examination.

Important Gems: Vitreoretinal Degeneration predisposing factors to a RD
1. **Lattice Degeneration:**
   Signs: Spindle-shaped, a network of white lines (can be pigmented) between the equator and the vitreous base posterior border. Small holes may be seen within the lattice. These are innocuous and commonly bilateral. They are usually present in 40% of patients with a Retinal Detachment, and there is an increased prevalence in myopic eyes.
2. **Snail Track Degeneration**
   Signs: Frost-like appearance, bands of tightly packed 'snowflakes' in the peripheral retina, white, can be longer than lattice degeneration, and round holes can form.
3. **White Without Pressure**
   Signs: Retina has a translucent grey appearance, linked to strong attachments to the vitreous gel, and giant tears can occur.
4. **Retinoschisis:** Splits or cysts within the neurosensory retina.
   Risk factor
   Proliferative Diabetic Retinopathy, vitreous traction and trauma.
   X linked: Women are usually carriers.
   Signs
   - Can cause reduced vision and peripheral/ absolute field defects, though often asymptomatic.
   - Cyst-like appearance.
   - Commonly bilateral and inferotemporal.
   - May find vitreous haemorrhages at the location of the cyst.

   Management
   A referral is necessary to confirm the diagnosis, then regular testing and monitoring for progression (1% progress to a Rhegmatogenous Retinal Detachment).

ADDITIONAL NOTES

3.9 VASCULAR OCCLUSIONS

Arterial Occlusions: Subdivided into Central and Branch Retinal Artery Occlusion

Risk Factor
- Age (increased risk after 50+) and a history of systemic vascular disease.

Symptoms

CRAO
- Sudden, painless, unilateral loss of vision.
- A ring of blindness that progresses inwards from the periphery towards the centre, can take two hours to progress/ notice upon waking. This is seen as a complete/ transient loss of vision or vision that resolves spontaneously **(Amaurosis Fugax)**.

BRAO
- Normal or reduced vision.
- Symptoms depend on how peripheral the occlusion is and whether it affects the temporal or nasal visual field. BRAO affecting the nasal visual field (temporal retina) may be asymptomatic due to the binocular overlap of the visual fields.
- A horizontal line of blindness sweeps up or down the VF but doesn't cross the H midline.

Signs

CRAO
- Reduced visual acuity (6/60 or worse). A patient may retain vision if a cilioretinal artery is present, supplying the macula.
- RAPD in the affected eye.
- Fundus: This may appear cloudy (yellow/ pale in appearance) in all quadrants.
- Disc oedema: This can occur a few hours after the initial onset of the condition.
- Cherry red spot at the macula.
- Arteries: Same colour and thickness as veins and narrow arterioles in all areas.
- Late stage of CRAO: Optic atrophy (no cupping, pale), cherry red spot disappears, and normal vessels are seen.

BRAO
- RAPD can be present.
- Fundus: The affected area of the fundus has a slightly yellow appearance.
- Sectoral optic atrophy.
- Lipid sheathing of the affected area and visible collateral shunt vessels.
- If the macula is involved, then vision is reduced.
- These patients can have an altitudinal or sectoral visual field loss.

Management
- An emergency referral to the cardiologist for a systemic workup.
- Timeframe of onset is important: First aid is necessary if the onset of the occlusion is less than 24 hours. This includes ocular massages and breathing into a paper bag.
  This is a rare condition but is extremely dangerous due to the threat to life and vision.

Prognosis
- **CRAO**: Approximately $1/3^{rd}$ of patients retain useful vision.
- **BRAO**: Most patients will have visual acuities of at least 6/12.
- Most patients will have a permanent visual field defect.
  To note: Neovascularization can occur within four weeks of an occlusion.
  The patient will report **reduced vision and a painful eye.**

Venous Occlusions: Subdivided into Central and Branch Retinal Vein Occlusion, which can be Ischaemic or Non-Ischaemic.

Risk factors
- Diabetes, Chronic Glaucoma, Atherosclerosis, cardiovascular disease, hypertension raised blood cholesterol, age, and a history of smoking.

Symptoms
- Painless, unilateral loss of vision or blurred vision.
- Often symptoms are noticed upon waking (Ask this specifically)

CRVO
- Normal or reduced (6/6 to CF).

BRVO
- Normal or sudden painless onset of blurred vision and metamorphopsia (if the macula is involved).
- Altitudinal visual field defect.

Signs

CRVO
- Disc and macula oedema.
- Haemorrhages (superficial, deep blot or flame-shaped). If haemorrhages are seen beyond the equator, this indicates primary Central Retinal Vein Occlusion.
- Intraretinal microvascular abnormalities (IRMA), dilated and tortuous veins.
- Cotton wool spots
  These signs may obscure the fundus view and are present in all four quadrants.

BRVO
- Occlusion commonly occurs at the A/V crossing.
- Haemorrhages (dot/ blot or flame-shaped) are commonly seen in the (ST) quadrant.
  These signs are only present in one quadrant.

Management
- Urgent referral to the GP for a systemic workup.
- Emergency to the casualty within 24 hours if there is a bilateral venous occlusion, the patient is young, IOP (> 40 mmHg), suspected angle-closure glaucoma or serious systemic disease.

Prognosis after 2-3months
- Non-ischaemic Vein Occlusion: Visual acuity improves (6/12 or better on the Snellen chart). Haemorrhages or oedema no longer remains.
- Ischaemic Vein Occlusion: Visual acuity remains reduced and may still have a RAPD.
- For Branch Retinal Vein Occlusion: Optociliary shunt vessels at the optic disc remain, and lipid/ fibrous sheathing of arteries and veins remain in the affected area.
- Neovascularization can occur: This can cause a RD, Neovascular Glaucoma and vitreous haemorrhage. Anterior segment neovascularization (e.g. Rubeosis Iridis) can occur from CRVO, and posterior segment neovascularization (e.g. new vessels at the disc/ elsewhere) more commonly occurs from BRVO or HRVO.

Differentiating between CRAO and CRVO
- ❖ **CRAO:** Severe vision loss, whitening of the retina and a cherry-red spot at the macula.
- ❖ **CRVO:** Reduced vision, haemorrhages in all four quadrants, cotton wool spots, exudates and new blood vessels.

Important Gems: How to distinguish between Ischaemic and Non-ischaemic Vein Occlusion.

Ischaemic Vein Occlusion
- Visual acuity 6/60 or worse (sudden vision loss, wavy lines reported in Amsler).
- RAPD is marked.
- Severe disc and macula oedema.
- Cotton wool spots, deep blot and flame-shaped haemorrhages.
- Severely tortuous and dilated veins.
- This condition can cause vitreous haemorrhage, Neovascular Glaucoma (rubeosis iridis), and Tractional Retinal Detachment.

Non-ischaemic Vein Occlusion
- Vision resolves itself, and 50% retain better than 6/60 on the Snellen chart.
- Mild or no disc and macula oedema.
- May have cotton wool spots, and tortuous/ dilated vessels.
- With or without a RAPD.

ADDITIONAL NOTES

3.10 OPTIC NEUROPATHY VS OPTIC NEURITIS

Optic Neuropathy: Subdivided into Arteritic and Non-arteritic Ischaemic Optic Neuropathy

1. **Giant cell Arteritis associated AION:** This is also known as Temporal arteritis.
Symptoms
- Headache (frontal/ temporal/ occipital/ generalised) exacerbates when lying down.
- Scalp tenderness, jaw pain (especially when chewing) and periocular pain.
- Diplopia
- The patient feels unwell.

Signs
- Sudden severe reduction in visual acuity.
- RAPD
- Fundus: Swollen discs that are pale and 'chalky white.'
    Cotton wool spots, splinter or flame-shaped haemorrhages.
- Third nerve palsy can occur.
- Visual field defect: central, paracentral, arcuate or altitudinal.

Management
- Emergency referral: If not done within this timeframe, the condition can occur in the second eye within two weeks. There is also a substantial risk of permanent vision loss and stroke due to the secondary association of AION; therefore, Giant Cell Arteritis is referred as an emergency.
    (Be cautious if an elderly patient complains of a recent headache or visual change and the signs above are noticed on examination).

2. **Arteritic Anterior Ischaemic Optic Neuropathy (AAION)**
Symptoms
- Diplopia, amaurosis fugax followed by a sudden severe loss of vision.
- Periocular pain.
- Symptoms usually reported by patients with Giant Cell Arteritis. Usually, this condition can occur within a few weeks of undiagnosed or untreated GCA.

Signs
- Severe reduction in visual acuity.
- Swollen discs: 'chalky white' and pale (a sign this is associated with GCA).

Management
- Emergency referral to prevent severe vision loss, blindness and second-eye involvement.

Non-arteritic Ischeamic Optic Neuropathy (NAION)
Symptoms
- Painless reduction in vision (within hours to days of initial onset or sudden decrease upon waking).
- Dyschromatopsia: This is proportionate to the level of visual impairment.
(This is a distinguishing factor to Optic Neuritis as colour is significantly affected and does not correlate to the level of VA reduction).

Signs
- Monocular loss in visual acuity.
- Fundus: Swelling of the optic nerve (diffuse or sectoral loss, without pallor initially) with or without splinter haemorrhages.
- Visual field defect. This is primarily an inferior altitudinal defect which causes an absolute scotoma; however, this can include central, paracentral or arcuate defects.

Management
- Referral to confirm the diagnosis and a GP referral for a systemic workup.

Optic Neuritis: Subdivided into Retrobulbar, Papillitis and Neuroretinitis

Symptoms
- Unilateral, progressive loss in vision (mild-severe) over a few days after the initial onset.
- Pain with eye movements in extreme gazes alongside eye and brow pain.
- Headache and tenderness of the globe.
- Dyschromatopsia: Colour is significantly affected and does not correlate to the level of VA reduction, e.g. mild loss in the visual acuity but a severe reduction in colour vision.
- The colour can appear washed out (red desaturation).
- Impaired night vision.
- Reduction in contrast, i.e. difficult to see words that are on a similar coloured background.
- Impaired depth perception: Difficult to judge distances when walking up and down stairs etc.

Signs
- Blurred or central VA loss with reduced contrast sensitivity; can be affected more with heat or exercise.
- Visual field loss: Central scotoma is common.
- RAPD if unilateral.
- Fundus: Swelling of the optic nerve that can be categorised into three types:
    1. **Retrobulbar**: Normal discs (pale in the early stages) and a miotic pupil (RAPD). This type of Optic Neuritis is associated with Multiple Sclerosis.
    2. **Papillitis**: Swollen discs with flame-shaped haemorrhages at the disc.
    3. **Neuroretinitis**: Papillitis and macula star (exudates in a star shape).

If the condition repeatedly occurs, Optic Neuritis can leave permanent damage resulting in optic atrophy.

Management
- Urgent or priority referral: Telephone the eye department for a triaged appointment.

Important Gem: Papilloedema
This term is exclusively used when disc swelling is secondary to intracranial pressure consisting of severe disc hyperaemia, blurred disc margins and disc elevation without a physiological cup. In addition, papilloedema is associated with brain tumours, idiopathic intracranial hypertension, central nervous system inflammation and cerebral venous thrombosis.

ADDITIONAL NOTES

3.11 UVEITIS

1. **Anterior Uveitis**
   - Iritis: Inflammation of the iris.
   - Iridocyclitis: Inflammation of the iris and pars plicata of the ciliary body.
2. **Intermediate Uveitis**
   - Inflammation of pars plana, the peripheral retina and the vitreous.
3. **Posterior Uveitis**
   - Choroiditis: Inflammation of the choroid.
   - Chorioretinitis: Secondary inflammation of the retina.
4. **Pan-Uveitis**
   - Combination of Anterior, Intermediate and Posterior Uveitis.

These inflammatory conditions are acute (sudden onset with a limited duration) or recurrent.

Acute Anterior Uveitis (AU)

Sx   Photophobia, dull aching pain (worse when reading/ accommodating), lacrimation and a red eye. (Episodes of ocular discomfort can occur a few days before the acute attack).

Signs
1. **Variable VA**: This depends on the severity of the inflammation. Usually, there is a mild reduction, but in severe cases of Anterior Uveitis, visual acuity can be 6/30 or worse.
2. **Anterior eye**: ciliary injection (ciliary flush) and conjunctival hyperaemia.
3. **Iris**: The presence of synechiae and/ or nodules, pupil block and iris bombé can occur. The risk of synechiae increases with a miotic pupil.
   - **Anterior synechiae**: Adhesions between the iris tissue and posterior corneal surface.
   - **Posterior synechiae**: Adhesions between inflamed iris tissue and the anterior surface of the crystalline lens.

   Nodules are usually seen in chronic cases of Anterior Uveitis.
   - **Koeppe nodules**: At the pupillary border, white and small in size.
   - **Busacca nodules**: Away from the pupil margins and within the iris stroma.
4. **Pupils**: Miotic, if severe, there will be a sluggish pupil response.
5. **Crystalline lens**: Pigment and fibrin deposits on the anterior surface and formation of PSC.
6. **Cornea**: Presence of keratic precipitates on the corneal endothelium.
   - Acute, non-granulomatous Anterior Uveitis: Fine, white KPs (milky spot appearance, triangular pattern and found inferiorly).
   - Chronic, granulomatous Anterior Uveitis: Generally large, yellow KPs (greasy looking, 'mutton fat' appearance, occurring in the lower third of the cornea). These may become pigmented with time.
7. **Anterior chamber**: white blood cells and hypopyon.
   Cells and flare (hazy appearance of the normally clear anterior chamber fluid).
   - (0) None, (1+) Faint 5-10 cells per field, (2+) Moderate 10-20 cells. Clear iris and lens detail, (3+) Marked 20-50 cells. Hazy iris & lens detail, (4+) Intense >50.
   - Hypopyon: Inflammatory cells, white, seen in the inferior portion of the AC. These are seen in severe cases of Anterior Uveitis, causing a severe reduction in vision.
8. **Anterior Vitreous**: If cells are detected in this location, suspect Posterior Uveitis.
9. **Retina**: Active or inactive inflammatory responses at the posterior pole or peripheral retina, Cystoid Macula Oedema and Posterior Uveitis in both eyes can be observed.

Management
    Refer   **Acute Uveitis:** Emergency referral to ophthalmic HES.
               Recurrent Uveitis (e.g. Iritis) Patient self-presents to HES when symptoms occur.
    Advice   Sunglasses for relief of acute symptoms of photophobia and discomfort.

Important Gems: Complications of Uveitis
1. Secondary Glaucoma: Blockage of the iridocorneal angle by cells causing IOP elevation.
2. Cataract: Direct onset due to inflammation and/or secondary to long-term steroid therapy.
3. Endophthalmitis: Intense inflammation of the entire eye.

Dilated fundus examination of both eyes is necessary when there is suspected Uveitis. This is to check for Cystoid Macula Oedema and Posterior Uveitis.

ADDITIONAL NOTES

3.12 BLEPHARITIS

Subdivided into Anterior and Posterior Blepharitis

<u>Anterior Blepharitis</u> **(Anterior Lid Margin Disease)**: Staphylococcal and Seborrhoeic
Cause: Infection, allergy, general sensitivity to bacteria on the eyelids and associated with some scalp conditions, e.g. oily skin, dry skin and dandruff.

<u>Posterior Blepharitis</u> **(Meibomian Gland Dysfunction)**
Cause: Blocked glands, unstable tear film, abnormal meibomian gland secretion and can be associated with patients who have acne rosacea.

A patient can present with the above or have a combination of both forms, as well as dry eye.

Risk factors
- Age and long-term contact lens wearer.

Symptoms
Asymptomatic or:
- Ocular discomfort (grittiness, burning, foreign body sensation)
- Sore or itchy lids
- Blurred vision
- Mild photophobia
- Symptoms similar to dry eye
- Contact lens intolerance

These symptoms are commonly bilateral, affecting both eyes symmetrically.

Signs
Staphylococcal Blepharitis
- Eyelashes: Misdirected, trichinosis, madarosis (loss of lashes).
- Eyelash roots: crustiness and white scales on the roots.
- Eyelid: Red, inflamed, crustiness of the lid margin and recurrent styes can be visible.
- Conjunctival hyperaemia and mild papillary Conjunctivitis can be observed.

Seborrhoeic Blepharitis
- Lid margins: Greasy appearance, hyperaemic, soft scales and lashes matted together.

Posterior Blepharitis
- Tear film: Oily, foamy or frothy appearance on the lid margin.
- Gland: gland loss, cystic dilatation or abnormal secretions.
- Posterior lid margin: hyperaemic.

Management: Regardless of the type of Blepharitis, the treatment remains the same.
1. Lid hygiene: Washing hands before and after cleaning the eyelids.
2. Warm compresses: Apply heat and massage.
3. Lid cleansing: Use sterile pads, individual moist wipes, cotton balls with separate cleaning solutions etc.
   - ❖ Gently rub the moistened pad or cotton ball along the upper and lower eyelid edges and wipe between the eyelashes. This is to remove any crusts and debris.
   - ❖ Repeat this process multiple times using a fresh pad/ wipe, then gently dry the eyes.
   - ❖ Duration: Twice a day for one month, then less often as it improves.
     Blepharitis is chronic in its clinical course, and lid cleansing should be done routinely to avoid flare-ups.
4. Treat any underlying dry eye if coinciding with Blepharitis.
5. Advice: Avoid rubbing your eyes and using cosmetics on the eyelid, e.g. eyeliner.
6. In severe cases: Antibiotic ointments are used, e.g. chloramphenicol, fusidic acid.
   Place into the eyes or rub into the lid margin with fingertips.

ADDITIONAL NOTES

3.13 CONJUNCTIVITIS

Subdivided into Infective, Allergic, Traumatic and Systemic.
Infective Three primary sources (bacteria, viruses, and other infective organisms).
Usually bilateral and contagious.
Allergic Two main types (atopic and non-atopic).
Traumatic Three primary sources (mechanical, chemical and radiation).
Systemic Rare but potentially the most serious.

Only the common subdivisions of Conjunctivitis will be discussed below.

Infective Conjunctivitis
1. Bacterial Conjunctivitis
Symptoms
- Reports exposure to an infected individual.
- Sore, gritty eyes, FB sensation and eyelids stuck together upon waking (lashes matted).
- Sticky discharge: Blurred transient vision if discharge crosses the pupil.

Signs
- The condition starts unilaterally but becomes bilateral within 1-2 days.
- Lid encrusting, lid inflammation and lash matting.
- Purulent/ mucopurulent discharge (an important sign this is bacterial).
- Diffuse conjunctival hyperaemia: maximum hyperaemia at the fornices.
- Mild papillary reaction: Solid areas of inflamed tissue around 0.2mm in diameter surrounding a central blood vessel at the tarsal conjunctiva.
- Diffuse corneal punctate epitheliopathy that stains with fluorescein.

Management
- Self-limiting within 5-7 days: Refer to GP within this timeframe for medical management to be of use, and broad-spectrum topical antibiotics for seven days are often prescribed.
- Refer if the condition fails to resolve or if there is a corneal involvement.
- Advice about personal hygiene: Avoid sharing towels and touching the eye, wash hands before handling food and use lid scrubs and eyewash. Cease contact lens wear until at least two days of complete resolution of the condition.

Associated Conditions
Bacterial Keratitis: To rule out this condition, look for corneal infiltration, ulceration and symptoms of photophobia or pain. If suspicious, an emergency referral is necessary.

2. Viral Conjunctivitis
Symptoms
- Reports exposure to an infected individual.
- Mild burning sensation in the eyes (as opposed to the gritty FB sensation in bacterial infections), mild photophobia, will often report flu-like symptoms and a sore throat.

To note: Vision will usually be unaffected.

Signs
- Condition starts unilaterally but becomes bilateral within 1-2 days.
- A watery discharge.
- Fine papillae
- Follicles are occasionally present at the tarsal conjunctiva and/ or lower fornix.
- Eyelid oedema and diffuse bulbar conjunctival injection (marked at the inner canthus).
- Pre-auricular lymph nodes may be tender (not always present).

To note: The pupil and cornea will not be affected.

Management
- Self-limiting within 1-2 weeks, cold compresses, hygiene measures (highly contagious, so avoid towel sharing and eye rubbing) and ocular lubricants for symptomatic relief.

Allergic Conjunctivitis (Atopic VS Non-Atopic)

Atopic Allergic Conjunctivitis

1. ***Seasonal Allergic Conjunctivitis (SAC)***
   As the allergen is pollen, signs and symptoms vary with the location, time of year (spring and summer), and weather conditions (maximal on high pollen count days).
   Symptoms
   - Itch
   - Report symptoms of sneezing and watery nasal discharge.
   - Family history and previous ocular history of the condition.

   Signs
   - A watery or mucous discharge with no pre-auricular lymph node swelling.
   - Diffusely oedematous conjunctiva, chemosis and lids can be swollen.
   - Papillary reaction: tarsal papillae (small, near fornices) and the tarsal conjunctiva has a velvety appearance.
   - Cornea: Uninvolved

   Management
   - Eyewash, cleaning the skin around the eye and cold compresses.
   - Topical antihistamines with ocular lubricants can provide temporary symptomatic relief.
   - Dual action mass cell stabilisers and antihistamines.
   - Advice: Avoid the allergen and excessively rubbing the eyes.

2. ***Perennial Allergic Conjunctivitis (PAC)***
   Cause: Allergenic material, e.g. household dust, animal fur, airborne moulds.
   Symptoms
   - Similar symptoms, signs, and management to Seasonal Allergic Conjunctivitis (SAC). The difference is symptoms can be all year round.

   Signs
   - Upper tarsal conjunctiva tends to be more affected than SAC.

   Management
   - Measures to avoid the allergen. These measures are more specialised for PAC, requiring special vacuum cleaner bags and bed linen.

Non-atopic Allergic Conjunctivitis (Contact Conjunctivitis)

Symptoms
- Report of a recent change, prolonged exposure to allergen placed directly in or near the eye, e.g. make-up, contact lens solution, therapeutic eye drops.
- Mild ocular pain and an itching sensation.
- Symptoms have built up gradually since the allergen first contacted the eye.

Signs
- Usually bilateral and symmetrical, but this also depends on the allergen.
- Watery or mucous discharge.
- Contact Dermatitis, e.g. facial rash around the eyes and lids.
- Tarsal conjunctival follicles and small papillae, e.g. mainly in the inferior fornix if therapeutic eye drops are the cause.
- Severe cases: Superficial corneal epithelial punctate staining with fluorescein and pre-auricular lymph nodes may be swollen.

Management
- Avoid the allergen and rubbing the eye excessively.
- Advice: Use ocular lubricants and cool compresses for symptomatic relief.

Traumatic Conjunctivitis

1. Mechanical Trauma – Giant Papillary Conjunctivitis (GPC)

Cause   The source and cause of the trauma will be known, e.g. contact lenses (non-disposable soft contact lens, RGP lenses), preservatives in the contact lens solution and ocular prosthesis.

Symptoms
- Itching (this may increase after lens removal), FB sensation and contact lens intolerance.
- Blurry vision (if there is mucous discharge).

Signs
- Stringy mucus discharge is found in the tear film or conjunctival surfaces. This can cause a reduction in visual acuity.
- Papillae: Micropapillae (0.3-1mm diameter in size) or giant papillae (>1mm diameter).
- Conjunctival oedema.
- Conjunctival hyperaemia.
- Upper tarsal conjunctiva is usually affected.
- In severe mechanical trauma, this can lead to lacerations or punctures.

(Even if signs are bilateral, they will be asymmetrical, as the condition is not due to, i.e. the lens itself, but a deposition causing the issues)

Management
- Management depends on the source and cause of the trauma. If it is related to contact lenses:
  - Replace soft lenses more frequently.
  - Optimise lens fit and material (fit those lenses that have better deposit resistance and/ or lower modulus).
  - Reduce wearing time or cease wear for a period.
- Improve hygiene: More rigorous surfactant cleaning.
- Pharmacological: Prescribe topical steroids, mast cell stabilisers and antihistamines.

2. Chemical Trauma

Signs and symptoms
- This can produce either Contact Allergic Conjunctivitis or a direct toxic effect.
- To note: If there is trauma to the globe and matter has flown into the eye, consider the possibility the globe has been penetrated and stain the eye to look for fluid leakage, e.g. in the case of welding.

3. Radiation Trauma

Symptoms
- Pain: Ranging from a mild foreign body sensation to intense pain.
- Tearing and reddening of the eye.
- A sensation of 'sand' in the eye.
- Abnormal sensitivity to light.

Signs
- This affects the conjunctiva and cornea simultaneously, as it is impossible to irradiate one without irradiating the other.
- Long-term effects of exposure, e.g. Cataract.

Conjunctivitis is a common acute side effect seen with chemical and radiation trauma. The signs, symptoms and management depend on the duration of exposure, intensity of the trauma/ radiation and the chemical/ radiation itself.

Important Gems: How to distinguish papillae from follicles.
Follicles
- Cystic in nature, translucent, less solid than papillae and have no central feeding blood vessel.
- Smooth, pale, pink-to-yellow, elevated lesions surrounded by displaced vessels.
- Generally seen in viral or chlamydial conditions.

Papillae
- Usually more discrete and redder than follicles.
- Contains a vascular core visible at the apex as a vascular tuft.

ADDITIONAL NOTES

3.14 DISORDERS OF THE CONJUNCTIVA/ SCLERA

Pinguecula

Cause Age and chronic exposure to dusty environments or to ultraviolet (UV) radiation.
Symptom
- Usually asymptomatic. If large, a pinguecula can interrupt the tear flow to the cornea, and patients then report ocular discomfort, e.g. a foreign body sensation.

Signs
- Raised area, yellow or white, translucent lesion, usually circular, commonly seen on the nasal side of the limbus.
- Corneal Dellen

Management
- Ocular lubricants are prescribed for symptomatic relief.
- Wrap-around sunglasses and hats: to prevent wind and exposure to ultraviolet radiation.

Surgery is not routinely advised to remove these lesions as they are benign.

Pterygium

Cause Due to chronic exposure to ultraviolet radiation, dryness, arid environment etc.
Symptoms
- Mild irritation and foreign body sensation. In some cases, patients are asymptomatic.

Signs
- Wing-shaped fibrovascular growth, can occur bilaterally but often asymmetrically.
- Usually on the nasal conjunctiva and close to the limbus.
- The pterygium can extend onto the cornea overlying the pupil. This is when vision is affected, and irregular astigmatism can occur.

Management
- Use a hat or wrap-around sunglasses: These measures protect against exposure to ultraviolet radiation, dust and wind, potentially decreasing the growth rate.
- Ocular lubricants advised for symptomatic relief.
- **Refer**: If there is a reduction in VA, irregular astigmatism or if it is cosmetically unappealing. Undergo surgical excision once growth extends and crosses the pupil area.
- **Advice**: Once grown, a pterygium will never reduce on its own.
  If surgically removed, a pterygium can regrow again.

Remember that two or more conjunctival conditions can co-exist. If in doubt, refer the patient for an ophthalmological opinion.

Subconjunctival Haemorrhage

Cause Spontaneous (after a cough or sneeze), straining, trauma (injury to the head), uncontrolled blood pressure and medication (warfarin, aspirin, NSAIDs etc.)
Sx Spontaneous redness with no report of pain, swelling or reduced vision.
Signs
- Unilateral
- Blood completely fills the clear space between the cornea and conjunctiva.

To eliminate other conditions, examine all extreme gazes whilst ensuring the posterior border is seen. If not seen, there is a possibility of an orbital fracture.

Management
- Self limiting within 1-2 weeks.
- If the condition reoccurs, refer to the GP for a systemic workup.

Episcleritis
Subdivided into Simple and Nodular Episcleritis.

Symptoms
- Redness, mild or dull pain (ache/ burning sensation, grittiness) and photophobia. (These symptoms occur acutely)

Signs
- Benign and usually recurrent.
- Sectoral hyperaemic injection, diffused or in one area (nodular), causing a mild elevation of the conjunctiva.

Simple Episcleritis
- VA is normal and usually bilateral.
- Sectoral redness or diffused.

Nodular Episcleritis
- This takes longer to resolve compared to Simple Episcleritis.
- A red, tender vascular nodule is observed.
- Other signs which can occur but are not common: elevated intraocular pressure (IOP) and an anterior chamber reaction.
  > To eliminate other conditions, the following must be normal: VA, palpebral conjunctiva, cornea, no discharge, no anterior chamber reaction.

Management
- Self-limiting (within 7-10 days, but this condition can last up to three weeks). If there is no improvement after three weeks, suspect a systemic involvement and refer to the hospital eye service (HES).
- For symptomatic relief: Cold compresses and ocular lubricants.
- Advice: This is a recurrent condition, to be aware if similar signs and symptoms occur and take appropriate steps to manage accordingly.

Differentiating between Scleritis and Episcleritis
Phenylephrine blanching technique: Use 2.5% or 10% concentration of phenylephrine to blanch the conjunctival and superficial episcleritis blood vessels. When deep episcleritis plexus does not blanch, this confirms the diagnosis of Scleritis. Vessels will blanch if the patient is suffering from Episcleritis.

Dry Eye
Subdivided into Aqueous Deficient or Evaporative Dry Eye.

Symptoms
- Asymptomatic or ocular irritation, foreign body sensation, gritty and burning sensation.

Signs — Exacerbated by smoke, wind, and heat.
- Usually bilateral.
- Lid wiper epitheliopathy.
- The Fl tear prism height on the inferior lid margin is less than 0.2mm.
- Reduced tear break up time (<10 seconds).
- With or without discharge: This can cause blurring of vision if there is a stringy mucous discharge or other tear film debris.

Management
- Educate the patient about the condition.
- Pharmacological: Ocular lubricants, ointments, or topical steroids.
- Tear conservation: Diminish outflow using punctal plugs.
- Deal with secondary causes, e.g. lid hygiene for meibomian dysfunction.

ADDITIONAL NOTES

3.15 CL ASSOCIATED INFILTRATIVE KERATITIS

Infiltrate VS Ulcer

Infiltrate
Cause A reaction to an immune response, e.g. contact lens-related cases (adverse reaction to the CLs material, over-wearing CLs), response to Viral Keratitis, pathogen on the lid margin etc.
Sx Asymptomatic or mild foreign body sensation.
Signs Small (< 2mm) and commonly located in the periphery.
Superficial staining with fluorescein.
(In majority of cases: there are no cells, lid involvement, discharge, or vision loss)

Ulcer
Cause Bacterial, Viruses (Herpes Simplex/ Herpes Zoster), Protozoa, Fungi, Autoimmune etc.
Onset Within 24 hours
Sx Photophobia, red eye, pain, teary eyes (lacrimation) and vision can be affected (if the ulcer is close to the visual axis).
Signs Large (>2mm), grey or white, dot-like appearance but can vary depending on the cause, epithelium and/or stromal stain with fluorescein (fuzzy edges) alongside conjunctival redness, the possibility of stromal oedema, discharge, lid swelling, ptosis, cells and flare.

Sterile Keratitis

1. Infiltrative Keratitis
Cause: An immune response.
Signs
- Corneal infiltrates, small sterile epithelial defects with or without an ulcer.
- Pannus (a small blood vessel that grows close to the infiltrate).

Management
- Self-limiting within 2-3 weeks.
- Can prescribe antibiotics or steroid drops for a faster recovery.

2. Contact Lens Induced Peripheral Ulcer (CLPU)
Sx Asymptomatic or photophobia, lacrimation, foreign body sensation and ocular discomfort.
Signs
- Pus discharge and conjunctival hyperaemia.
- Ulcer located in the periphery but if central <2mm in size. *(No cells will be present)*

Management
- Self-limiting: Most signs and symptoms relieve after 48 hours.
- Advice: To temporally cease contact lens wear.
- It is important to monitor for 24 hours (refer if there is any suspicion of an infected ulcer).

Marginal Keratitis

Cause Bacterial, upper respiratory tract infection etc.
Sx The severity of pain varies from ocular discomfort to foreign body sensation, photophobia, teary eyes (lacrimation) and a red eye. The patient may report recurrent episodes.
Signs
- Ulcer/ infiltrate, white, round or curved, bulbar conjunctiva can be hyperaemic and oedematous, circumlimbal injection and signs of Blepharitis can be visible too.

Management
- Self-limiting; however, use ocular lubricants or topical antibiotics for symptomatic relief.
- Advise using sunglasses for acute photophobic symptoms and lid hygiene for any associated Blepharitis. If the condition is recurrent, refer to the hospital eye service (HES).

Microbial Keratitis: Infected Ulcer

1. Bacterial Keratitis

Symptoms
- Photophobia, blurred vision, purulent or mucopurulent discharge.

Signs
- Variable signs depending on the severity and cause of the condition.
- Ranges from infiltrates causing an epithelial defect, stromal oedema, circumcorneal injection and eyelid swelling to scarring, ulceration and secondary conditions such as Anterior Uveitis, Endophthalmitis etc.

2. Viral Keratitis: Herpes Simplex Keratitis and Herpes Zoster ophthalmicus

Herpes Simplex Keratitis

History of a cold or flu-like symptoms.
The patient reports recurrent cold sores (Optometrist may see a cold sore on examination).

Symptoms
- The severity of the symptoms varies. Symptoms can decrease with an increased number of episodes.
- Pain (burning, irritation), photophobia, reduced vision and lacrimation.

Signs
- Cornea: Large dendritic ulcer/s
  Four types
  1. **Epithelial:** Dendritic ulcer/s.
  2. **Stromal**: Infiltrates, vascularisation, keratic precipitates (KP) with raised intraocular pressure, secondary conditions such as Uveitis etc.
  3. **Disciform keratitis**: Folds in the Descemet's membrane, KP and Uveitis.
  4. **Metaherpetic ulcer**: Trophic Keratitis.

Management
- Refer as an emergency when:
  1. The stroma is involved
  2. The condition is bilateral affecting both eyes.
  3. The patient is young.
  4. The patient is a contact lens wearer.
- Monitor for 72 hours without referring if this is a recurrent episode and the stroma is not involved.
- Refer urgently (within one week) if the epithelium has not healed within seven days.
  (If not treated appropriately, this condition can lead to a geographic/ amoebic ulcer).

Herpes Zoster ophthalmicus

Symptom and signs
- Acute phase: Discomfort, teary eyes (lacrimation), pain, photophobia, discharge and redness.
- Hutchingson sign: Lesion on the tip of the nose (indicating an ocular involvement).
- Complications and secondary conditions associated:
  Keratitis, Episcleritis, Scleritis, Conjunctivitis, Anterior Uveitis, Secondary Glaucoma.
  This can occur months to years after the acute phase.

Management
- Self-limiting within 10-14 days, even if left untreated.
- Symptomatic relief: Cold compresses, ocular irrigation and ocular lubricants.
- Refer to the GP for prophylactic antibiotic therapy.

3. Protozoal: Acanthamoeba

Symptoms
- Moderate to severe eye pain and photophobia (no relief even after contact lens removal).
- The patient may report poor contact lens hygiene, recent corneal trauma or water exposure (swims/ showers with their contact lenses and/ or cleans lenses/ case with tap water).

Signs
- Signs are not proportionate to the symptoms reported (mild signs but symptoms are severe)
- Visual acuity reduction (at least by two lines on the Snellen chart).
- Lid oedema and discharge.
- A large ulcer, central to the visual axis, and the stroma is involved.
- Cells, flare and hypopyon.

This condition can be difficult to diagnose. In the initial stages, the signs are mild and may resemble Viral Conjunctivitis, and then it can appear like Herpes Simplex Keratitis. If still not managed accordingly, this can progress to stromal penetration with anterior cells, flare and hypopyon.

Management
- Emergency referral to the HES. Advise the patient to take their contact lens case with them.

Important Gems:
Viral conditions are highly contagious (do not share towels etc.)
Wash hands before and after the examination and clean equipment rigorously before the next patient.

ADDITIONAL NOTES

BINOCULAR VISION ABNORMALITIES

4.1 MUSCLE INACTION

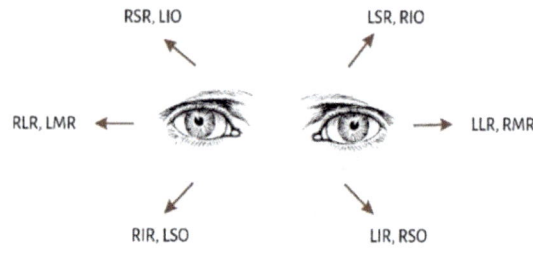

Lateral Rectus (LR)
- **Greatest defect**: When abducting (out) the paretic eye.
- Primary position: Esotropia (usually)
- Head position: Towards the palsied side.

Superior Rectus (SR)
- **Greatest defect**: In elevation and abduction (out) of the paretic eye but normal on adduction (in).
- Primary position: Paretic eye is hypotropic.

Medial Rectus (MR)
- **Greatest defect**: When adducting (in) the paretic eye.
- Primary position: Exotropia
- Head position: Towards the sound side.

Inferior Rectus (IR)
- **Greatest defect**: In downward gaze when abducting (out) the paretic eye.
- Primary position: The unopposed antagonist (SR) causes the paretic eye to be incyclotropic and hypertropic.
- Head position: Downwards, to the paretic side, with a tilt to the sound side.

Superior Oblique (SO)
- **Greatest defect**: When adducting in depression.
- Primary position: Overaction of the antagonist (IO), causing the paretic eye to be hypertropic.
- Head position: Tilted towards the uninvolved side, and the chin is depressed.

Inferior Oblique (IO)
- **Greatest defect**: In upward gaze when adducting (in) the paretic eye. Overaction of the unopposed antagonist (SO) will cause incyclotropia.
- Head position: Head inclined towards the paretic side and face turned towards the sound side.

(Least likely of the muscles innervated by the third cranial nerve to be paralysed, and often confused with Browns Tendon Sheath Syndrome).

4.2 INCOMITANCE

Concomitant: A tropia/phoria that is constant regardless of the fixating eye or direction of gaze.
Incomitant: A tropia/ phoria that changes in magnitude depending on the fixating eye or direction of gaze.
- If recent onset: An abnormal head posture (AHP) can be observed, but once the affected eye is occluded, the AHP will no longer be present. Also, the onset of symptoms will be known.
- If longstanding: Intermittent and less marked due to progressive comitancy and suppression. The patient may not complain of symptoms, and there will be no diplopia unless the affected eye decompensates. The patient may have an AHP, and even after occluding the affected eye, this will make no difference.

Abnormal Head Posture
- Face turn to right/ left: Anomaly of the medial rectus/ lateral rectus.
  The face will turn towards the affected muscle, e.g. LLR palsy, with face turn to the left.
- Chin elevation or depression: This is usually seen in Brown syndrome.
- Head tilt: There can be a combination of head tilt, face turn and chin elevation/ depression.
- The absence of an abnormal head posture does not mean an absence of incomitancy. An abnormal head posture can sometimes remain simply due to habit.

(Diplopia is common upon straightening the head or tilting to the opposite side. The head may also straighten when the eye with the paretic muscle is occluded).

Muscle Sequele
Four stage process after the onset of a palsy
1. Underaction of the primary muscle   e.g.   **RSR**
2. Overaction of the contralateral synergist   **LIO**
3. Overaction of the ipsilateral antagonist   **RIR**
4. Underaction of the contralateral antagonist   **LSO**

Incomitant Nerve Palsy
Signs and symptoms vary depending on if the condition is recently acquired or is long-standing.
Symptoms: The patient usually reports difficulty looking towards a particular gaze position.
Signs: An abnormal head posture is present (face turn/ chin elevation or depression/ head tilt).

Sixth Nerve Palsy   **EOM: Lateral Rectus affected**
- **Common cause**: Multiple Sclerosis, Hypertension, Diabetes, Trauma etc.
- **Signs**: The patient cannot move their eye to the temporal side; therefore, the primary position is affected, and the eye turns **in**.
  For long-standing sixth nerve palsies: There is normal adduction with limited abduction of the affected eye. This is more prominent when the patient looks at a distant target and less obvious or minimal for near targets.

Fourth Nerve Palsy   **EOM: Superior Oblique affected**
- **Common cause**: Trauma, congenital, microvascular disease or idiopathic
- **Signs**: Ipsilateral hypertropia and excyclotorsion. May develop a head tilt.

Third Nerve Palsy   **Superior-SR, inferior-MR, IR, IO**
- **Common cause**: Trauma, Tumour, Diabetes, Hypertension etc.
- **Signs**: The affected eye is **down and out,** ptosis, mydriasis, paresis of accommodation and loss of pupil action (fixed, dilated pupils)

Important Gems: Acquired Third Nerve Palsy and RAPD
Assume this is due to an aneurysm unless proven otherwise.

ADDITIONAL NOTES

ACCURATE RECORDING AND ANALYSIS

5.1 H&S SIGHT TEST
Appropriate questions and how to record (in blue) the patient's response.

RFV: Are you having any problems with your eyes, or is this a routine check-up?
LEE: x/24, routine   (Investigate with LOFTSEA for all symptoms reported)
No headaches, no flashes, no floaters, no diplopia, no red eye, and no problems reported.
                (Negative marking is important and must be included in the record)
Current Rx: Do you have glasses? How many? Type? (SV/ Bifocal/ Varifocal) Any coating/ tint?
How old are your current glasses? Constant wear or occasional wear?
Are you happy with your glasses regarding fit? Fashion? Vision?
C Rx   DV: Good, NV: Good, INT: Good (Specify the preferred working distance)
S Rx   DV: Good, NV: Good
Whilst reading, are you holding the book at your preferred distance for near or further away?
                (Tailor the question to the patient and their preferred task and distance).
Contact lens: What type? (Daily/ Monthly lenses) Last aftercare? Who supplied them?
Is your vision good with CLs? Are you happy with the level of vision in your lenses?
Is your vision similar to spectacles?

OH: Have you ever seen a specialist/ HES for your eyes? If so, who referred you? Clinic name?
Any treatment? Last and next check-up? Discharged and when?
No Glaucoma   (Open/ Closed), (1/ both eyes) Age of onset? Any previous treatment?
No Cataract   (1/ both eyes). Age of onset?
No Amblyopia   Which eye? Any previous treatment, e.g. spectacles prescribed/ patching/ surgery?

GH: Last medical examination, and what was the outcome?
       Any previous or current treatment?
No Diabetes   (Type 1/ 2) Good control? If so, how? By diet/ tablets/ insulin?
                Last diabetic screening test? Specialist's name? The outcome of the examination?
No Hypertension Good control? When was your last blood pressure check-up?
Medication: None (Name of drug, dose and frequency) Onset?
Any Allergies?
Smoker: Yes/ no

FOH: Is there anyone in the family with an eye condition?
No Glaucoma   (Type). Age when the patient was diagnosed and onset.
No Amblyopia.   (Specifically ask this question when testing a child)
FGH
No Diabetes

HOBBIES: Swim (Do you wear goggles/ CLs?), Read (c/s Rx), Sports (Do you wear safety Rx?)
VDU: How many hours in a day? (x/24, c/ s Rx?) Regular breaks? Any specific add for VDU use?
Any headaches or symptoms whilst using VDU? Do the symptoms increase in the evening?
OCCUPATION: Is any specific Rx required for work? (Occupational lenses/ safety Rx/ CLs)
DRIVE: Yes/ no/ learning to drive
       (Vehicle type, e.g. HGV) Do you wear Rx whilst driving? Drive at night? Glare symptom?

Concluding question at the end: "Would you like to add anything I may have forgotten?"

LOFTSEA

Location:	R/ L/ BE/ Diffused area/ Location on the head/ Position of gaze (for diplopia)
Onset:	When did it start? / Sudden or gradual start? Time of day? Duration?
Frequency:	How often does it occur? Is there a pattern?
Type:	Constant, or does it come and go? Has this happened before?
Self-relief:	Better or worse with a specific task, e.g. computer/ resting.
Effect on the patient:	What does it prevent you from doing?
	If severe, have you seen a specialist/ HES about it?
Associated factors:	Are there any other symptoms associated with this?

LOFTSEA For Specific Symptoms

1. *Headache*
   - Location of the headache (frontal/ parietal/ occipital area).
   - Pain (throbbing/ sharp/ dull ache). How severe is the pain from 1-10?
   - Worse when bending down?   (Can be linked with sinusitis)
   - Worse at the end of the day? Better during weekends? Do you wear up-to-date Rx?

   (Can be linked with Asthenopia)

2. *Diplopia*
   - Monocular (clarify which eye)/ binocular? With or without Rx?
   - Position of gaze (H/ V/ In all directions), any changes since the onset? Occur when tired?
   - Does it disappear if you cover one eye?   (If yes, can be linked to a BV issue)
   - Previous history of diplopia? Normal birth history?

3. *Dry eyes*
   - Watery?
   - Photophobia? Blurred vision?
   - Do symptoms improve after blinking?
   - Any symptoms whilst reading? Any symptoms whilst using VDU?
   - Specific times when the dry eye is worse, e.g. windy conditions, whilst driving, using air conditioning?

4. *Red eye*
   - Constant redness or intermittent?
   - Discharge? Any associated pain?
   - Have you suffered from any recent illnesses?
   - Family member with a recent red eye?
   - Any allergies? Any back pain? Arthritis?
   - Has this ever happened before? If so, what was said? Did you see a specialist? Was any medication given?
   - Do you wear contact lenses? Do you sleep, shower or swim with your lenses? Do you clean your contact lens or case with tap water?

5. *Floater*
   - Onset?
   - Appearance? How many? Colour?
   - Constant or intermittent?
   - Any flashing lights or curtain in your vision?
   "If you look at a uniformed background, do the floaters move down with gravity?"

USEFUL EARLY RETEST NHS CODES

1.	At risk of frequent Rx changes that do not require a medical referral.
2.	Suffering from an ocular condition that is likely to worsen, e.g. Cataract.
3.	Signs and symptoms that require ophthalmic investigation resulting in: 3.1: A referral to the GP/ medical professional. 3.2: A new prescription for spectacles. 3.3: No change in spectacles or a referral. (Ensure the records indicate symptoms suggesting the necessity for an early sight test)
4.	4.1: Requiring complex lenses. 4.2: Best corrected visual acuity of 6/60 or worse in one eye.
5.	5.1: GP/ medical professional has requested the patient to have a sight test. 5.2: The patient is being investigated by an Optometrist (with the required qualifications). 5.3: Seen more frequently due to risk factors identified in protocol.
6.	Anything else that is unusual requiring a clinical investigation and does not meet the above standards.

SUPPLEMENTARY CODES

2.0	Following on from a sight test, carrying out a cycloplegic refraction.
2.1	Paediatric follow-up.
2.2	Referral refinement, repeat or follow-ups.
2.3	Suspect glaucoma patient.
2.4	<60 dilation & biomicroscopy.
2.5	Anterior segment disorders.
2.6	Cycloplegic refraction was requested by the hospital eye service (HES).
2.7	Postoperative Cataract examination.

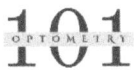

5.2 REFERRAL LETTER TEMPLATE

Date: Optometrist's Name   ………………..
Name of Consultant   ……………………   Practice Address   ………………..
Hospital Address   ……………………   Telephone Number   ………………..

Patient's Name   ……………………….
Patients D.O.B   ………………………

Reason For Referral

………………………………………………………………………………………………………

………………………………………………………………………………………………………

………………………………………………………………………………………………………

The patient attended a routine/ early sight test complaining of ………………………………………..
(Do LOFTSEA on the symptoms reported and relate it to the tentative diagnosis)

On examination:

Results ……...……………………………………………………………………………………..
VA
IOP
Visual field
Refraction
Other tests …….…………………………………………………………………………………….
(Record any relevant tests and results based on what you suspect is the tentative diagnosis)

Referral as ……………………….. to …….………………………….. (Indicate the timeframe)
A letter was sent to the GP to inform them.
(Here, you can write your tentative diagnosis, but if you record accurately, it should be obvious what the tentative diagnosis is).

If you require further information, please do not hesitate to contact me.
Kind regards,

……………………………………….
(Optometrist's name and signature)

5.3 H&S CONTACT LENS AFTERCARE

Appropriate questions and how to record (in blue) the patient's response.

Patient's Name ....
Date and Time ....
Reason For Visit: Aftercare/ Specific problem?

Ask open questions (Investigate with *LOFTSEA*)

Symptoms
No Headaches
No Lacrimation (Do you have teary eyes?)
No Photophobia (Do you have any sensitivity to light?)
(Negative marking is important, include it in the record)
Comfort: Good. Any discomfort with the contact lens? Grittiness?
   Is there a drop in comfort from the start to the end of the month? (Monthly CLs)
   Do your eyes get tired by the end of the day? End of the wearing time?
   Any dry eye symptoms?
VA: D/N Good with contact lens. Any blur?

Current Contact Lens Specification
(R/L) Manufacturer's name: BC/ TD/ Rx. Details of modality and material.
E.g. RE, Maxim: Soft SiH daily lens 8.14: 14.2: +1.75

Contact Lens History
Previous contact lens details: Any changes to the current lenses worn? If so, why did you change?
   Which contact lens solution do you use?
Last Aftercare: x/24
Last Eye Test: x/24. Do you have backup spectacles? Good vision with Rx for all tasks.
   Is the vision in your lenses just as good as your spectacles?
Wearing time: Today (x/24), average (x/24) and maximum (x/24).
   How many times do you wear your contact lenses during the week?

Compliance
1. Do you swim, shower or sleep in your lenses?
2. Describe the care routine. If ok, record 'care routine good'.
3. If wearing monthly lenses: How do you clean your lenses? How do you store your lenses?
   How often is the case changed?

OH: No HES, no eye problems. History of any infections?
GH: No Diabetes, no hypertension, no cold sores.   Allergies: None
   Medication: (Name of drug, dose and quantity) Onset? Reason for use?
FOH/ FGH

Hobbies
Occupation
Smoker: Yes/ no
VDU: How many hours (x/24) in a day? With or without Rx? Regular breaks?
   Is any specific Rx used?
Drive: Yes/ no / learning to drive
   Do you wear Rx whilst driving? Do you drive at night? Any glare symptoms?

Concluding question: 'Would you like to add anything I may have forgotten?'
Lastly, observe the general blink rate. If the patient blinks excessively, this suggests a shorter tear break-up time (TBUT).

5.4 CL TESTS AND APPROPRIATE RECORDING

First Choice Soft Contact Lens Specification
1. **BOZR**: Flattest K (biggest number) + (0.7-1.00)
    - Too tight: Increase BOZR by 0.5
    - Too loose: Decrease BOZR by 0.5
2. **Total diameter:** HVID (mm) + 2mm as a guide.
   A cornea with a large HVID needs a flatter lens, and a small HVID needs a steeper lens.
3. **Power**: Sphere + ½ cyl
   If astigmatism is > 1.00DC, check cross cyl and order toric contact lens.
   Axis: Use the spectacle prescription axis.
4. Other necessary measurements: PA size and pupils in low light.

To determine contact lens modality and type, always consider the wearing time.
For example, a tight-fitting contact lens may be acceptable for a wearing time of 2-3 hours but may not be accepted if the same fit is seen but the wearing time is 12 hours.

Tests to determine the most appropriate CLs
1. **Measure distance/ near visual acuity**
2. **Over refraction**
   Firstly using best vision sphere (BVS), followed by binocular over-refraction, +1.00 blur test and then determine the final VA.
   - Tight-fitting CLs: Will give an unreliable over-refraction.
   - Loose-fitting CLs: Will give a variable over-refraction, and the prescription changes each time.
3. **Check D/N visual stability:** Check if vision is stable and clear after blinking.
   Procedure: Ask the patient to focus on a letter and then blink. (Repeat this with a near target)
   Question: After the blink, is the letter the same, clearer or does it go blurry?
   - Tight-fitting CLs: The letter is **clearer** after the blink.
   - Loose-fitting CLs: The letter is **blurry** after the blink.
4. **Check Lens Stability**: Check if there is a crisp neutralised reflex with and without blinking on retinoscopy.
   - Tight-fitting CLs: Poor retinoscopy reflex with distortions.
   - Loose-fitting CLs: Clear reflex centrally and distorted peripherally.
         (Some lenses, e.g. thin conventional hydrogels do not show this)
5. **On CLs removal**
   Tight-fitting CLs: Causes compression of the limbal conjunctiva.
   Loose-fitting CLs: Causes buckling of the lens edge.

Recording the Contact Lens Fit
1. Centration: Position and if acceptable, e.g. fully centred/ 0.5mm inferiorly but acceptable.
2. Coverage: Full coverage over the cornea in all positions of gaze. Does not cross the limbus.
3. Diameter: Big/ small. Off to one side by (x)mm but acceptable/ not acceptable.
4. Post blink: Patient looks up and then blinks, then down and blinks, then to each side and blinks.
    - Record: Good movement with blink.
    - Post blink: Normal values are between 0.2-0.4.
        (< 0.2 is tight/ inadequate movement and > 0.4 is loose/ excessive movement)
    - H lag: Fast and smooth, slow and jerky etc.
5. Push-up test: Patient looks straight ahead. Push the CLs up and let the lens come down whilst observing. Record 'Easy to push up, smooth and quick recovery/ slow and sluggish recovery'.
6. Summary of fit: 'As patient wears for (x)hours, this fit is acceptable/ not acceptable'.
   Include a summary based on the lens condition and previous points, e.g. centration, coverage.

Post Contact Lens Examination
Below is an example of how to record a normal, healthy eye when using slit lamp Biomicroscopy. Use this as a guide but always record any abnormalities seen. Assess & record RE/LE separately.

Lids	Clear, no Blepharitis or blocked glands, punctum open and clear.
Grading	Write down which chart was used, e.g. Efron.
	❖ Grade lid roughness
	❖ Grade hyperaemia: limbal, bulbar and palpebral conjunctiva.
	❖ Draw or describe hyperaemia, superficial staining and any signs of neovascularisation.
Iris	No pigment change.
Sclera	White
Cornea	Clear/ no corneal staining.
Lens	Clear and transparent.
Vitreous	Uniform background.
Anterior Chamber	
	Grade using Van Herricks. Also, record 'no anterior chamber cells or flare'.

Common findings when wearing poorly fitted contact lenses
- Scratched epithelium
- Punctate staining: This can also suggest incomplete blinking if seen inferiorly.
- Limbal indentation (fluorescein pooling): Seen after immediately removing the soft contact lens and when the fit is tight.
- Ring of staining around the conjunctiva: Due to silicone hydrogel abrasions of high modulus lens material or when lenses are drying out. This is a sign of an unacceptable fit.

Tear Tests
- Keratometer: NIBUT and mire quality (normal TBUT is 15+ seconds).
- Tear prism: Normal/ 0.2 central, 0.1 peripheral.
- Tear viscosity, debris, blink rate and lid tension: Record 'normal/ good'.
      Describe the appearance if abnormal.

Management of Contact Lens Associated Symptoms
In some cases, presenting symptoms can be linked to poor compliance and the contact lens itself rather than an underlying ocular disease. Therefore an Optometrist must eliminate some of these causes by managing the symptoms before considering a differential diagnosis of ocular pathology.

Dry Eye Symptoms
- Advise on using artificial drops during the day as and when required.
- Refit with daily contact lens if they are wearing monthly or extended-wear lenses.
- Fit with silicone hydrogel contact lens as it dehydrates less.
- When using VDU, take regular breaks.
- Check if the patient blinks appropriately and completely. If not, advise blinking exercises.

Corneal Staining with Fluorescein
- Increase Dk/t and change the solution used.
- Prescribe artificial tears, check if the patient blinks completely and advise on blinking exercises.
- Cease or decrease wearing time to 3-4 hours, then increase gradually in small increments.

Reduced Vision and Astigmatism
- Prescribe Toric SiH/ RGP lenses.

Poor Compliance
- Re-educate on hygiene, lens care and case care (replace every month, rinse and dry daily).
- Reinforce not to swim, shower or sleep in their contact lens.

Important Gems: If the contact lens chosen is suitable yet symptoms remain unexplained, dwell deeper into pathological causes and ocular diseases.

ADDITIONAL NOTES

5.5 VISUAL FIELD ANALYSIS
Based on the acronym 'WANDER'.

(W) Which technique was used?
Record the visual field machine, degree and strategy, e.g. Henson, 24-2, supra threshold.

(A) How accurate are the results?
Repeat if the value for false positive (FP) is >15% or fixation losses are 20%.
Other causes affecting data: Not inputting or using the patient's correct prescription.
Artefacts due to spectacle rim, droopy lids, brow and lashes.

(N) Is the field normal? Always input the patient's date of birth into the visual field machine.
1. Total Deviation (TD): Normal (+ or – 2DB)
   - A negative value means the sensitivity is lower than normal. A high negative value means the patient requires a brighter than normal stimulus to see, indicating the visual field is getting worse.
   - A positive value means the sensitivity is higher than normal.
2. Mean Deviation (MD): Normal (0 to -2db)
   This value evaluates the overall sensitivity of the field, comparing the results to the age-matched normal. An average value of total deviation (TD) is used, but there is an emphasis on the central area. Media opacities can affect the results too. A high negative value indicates a brighter light is required to see the target.
3. Pattern Standard Deviation (PSD): Normal is between 0 to 4.
   - Cataract/ small pupils do not affect the results as diffused loss is removed. This allows a distinction between localised defects that are disease-related and media opacities.
   - PSD is affected by FP and FN results which can give false readings if undetected.
4. P value: Anything other than zero is abnormal.
   This value highlights the probability of an abnormal value occurring in a normal patient.
5. Glaucoma Hemifield Test: Judges the overall symmetry of sensitivity of 5 areas in the superior and inferior field. If there is an asymmetry in the H midline, this is a sign of Glaucoma.
6. Greyscale plot: This gives a general idea of the location and size of a defect. Darker areas are problem areas. A 'clover leaf defect' is seen when a patient is tired or is a sign of early disease.

(D) If abnormal, what defects are present?
Confirm: Which eye? Where (S/I/ T/ N)? Same side or the opposite side?
Describe the defect:
- Defects are either focal (in one area) or diffused.
- Paracentral defect (close to centration) or an enlarged blind spot.
- Arcuate: Elongating paracentral defect yet still respecting the horizontal midline.
- Nasal step: There is a difference above and below the horizontal midline in the nasal field, and it is associated with differences in the sensitivity of the retina.

(E) Evaluate the field: Compare the field plots based on disc appearance. Always check if it correlates to the VF defect, e.g. inferior NRR thinning will cause a superior visual field loss.

(R) Is the field repeatable?

1.	Early	MD > -6db
		5% probability level defect for < 18 of tested points
		1% < 10 of tested points
2.	Moderate	MD -6db > -12db
		5% probability level defect for < 37 of tested points.
		1% < 20 of tested points
		Sensitivity <15db in central 5 degrees on only one hemifield.
3.	Advanced	MD -12db > -20
		5% probability level defect for > 37 of tested points.
		1% > 20 of tested points
		Sensitivity <15db in central degrees on both hemifields.

5.6 WHERE IN THE VISUAL PATHWAY?

With a visual field plot, you can determine where in the visual pathway an issue occurs. There are specific characteristics you should consider for an accurate diagnosis.

Abnormalities at the:
1. **Optic nerve**: Can cause a **Monocular** defect/ **RAPD**/ VA and colour reduction.
   If a visual field (VF) defect represents V midline: It is due to a neurological issue.
   If a VF defect represents H midline: Due to a retinal nerve fibre defect (Glaucoma) or vascular problem (vascular occlusions/ NAIO etc.)
2. **Chiasm**: **Binocular (heteronymous)** defect/ **RAPD**/ normal or reduced VA and colour.
   - Bitemporal VF defect (e.g. pituitary gland tumour).
   - Binasal VF defect (e.g. ophthalmic artery supplying the nerve dies, causing ischaemic optic neuropathy/ aneurysm in the post-communicating artery).
3. **Optic tract**: Binocular **homonymous** hemianopia (same side)/**non-congruous** defect/ RAPD
   e.g. RHS homonymous hemianopia affects the L optic tract (LHS of the brain).
4. **LGN**: Homonymous hemianopia/ RAPD
   e.g. RHS homonymous hemianopia affects L LGN.
   (After the LGN: No RAPD is present)
5. **Optic radiation**: Homonymous **quadranopia** and normal pupils.
   - Pie in the sky
     e.g. Superior Homonymous quadranopia due to damage to the inferior optic radiation in the temporal lobe.
   - Pie on the floor
     e.g. Inferior homonymous hemianopia due to damage to the superior optic radiation in the parietal lobe.
6. **Visual cortex**: **Congruous**, homonymous hemianopia with **macula sparing**.
   e.g. R homonymous hemianopia with macular sparing affects L visual cortex.

Defects in Glaucoma
1. Early relative or arcuate defect. The first sign is a superior nasal (SN) visual field defect which correlates to inferior temporal (IT) neuroretinal rim loss.
2. Paracentral defect: Defect close to centration.
3. Absolute defect: Does not cross the horizontal midline and may cause an enlarged blind spot.
4. Nasal step
5. Multiple arcuate defects: Peripheral breakthrough and a threat to fixation.
6. End-stage: Results in a temporal island.

Important Gems
1. **Visual Field Plot:** The location of the blind spot corresponds to the eye
   e.g. for the right eye (RE), the blind spot is on the right-hand side (RHS).
2. **Fundus Photo:** The location of the optic nerve corresponds to the eye
   e.g. for the right eye (RE), the optic nerve is on the right-hand side (RHS).
3. **Volk:** Use the macula as a guide to reference where a lesion is.
   Remember, the macula is always on the temporal side, and the image is inverted (S/ I).
   - If you see a defect that is above the optic nerve and closer to the optic nerve (compared to the macula), in reality it is inferior nasal (IN).
   - If you see something above the macula, close to the macula, in reality, it is (IT).
   - If you want to see the superior fundus, ask the patient to look up and tilt the volk lens upwards slightly. The image will be inferior when viewed with a volk lens.

Important Gems:
Suppose a patient has a Homonymous Hemianopia (HH); in that case, they have reasonable distance and near vision but may complain whilst reading, e.g. Left HH struggle to start reading sentences, and Right HH struggle to read the end of sentences.

ADDITIONAL NOTES

ADDITIONAL NOTES

ABBREVIATIONS

AACG	Acute Angle Closure Glaucoma	LHS	Left-Hand Side
AC	Anterior Chamber	LME	Last Medical Examination
AC/A	Convergence induced by accommodation per Dioptre of accommodation	LR	Lateral Rectus
		LVA	Low Vision Aid
AHP	Abnormal Head Posture	MD	Macular Degeneration
AION	Arteritic Ischaemic Optic Neuropathy	MR	Medial Rectus
AMD	Age-Related Macular Degeneration	MS	Multiple Sclerosis
AS	Anterior Scleritis	NPC	Near Point of Convergence
A/V	Arteriovenous	NRR	Neuroretinal Rim
BDR	Background Diabetic Retinopathy	NTG	Normal Tension Glaucoma
BOZR	Back Optic Zone Radius	NV	Near Vision
BRAO	Branch Retinal Arterial Occlusion	NVD	New Vessel at Disc
BV	Binocular Vision	NVE	New Vessel Elsewhere
C	With	ONH	Optic Nerve Head
CCT	Central corneal thickness	PAC	Perennial Allergic Conjunctivitis
CF	Count Fingers	PCO	Posterior Capsular Opacification
CLs	Contact Lenses	PVD	Posterior Vitreous Detachments
CRAO	Central Retinal Artery Occlusion	PS	Posterior Scleritis
CS	Contrast sensitivity	PSC	Posterior Subcapsular Cataract
CWS	Cotton Wool Spots	Px	Patient
C/D	Cup-to-disc ratio	RAPD	Relative Afferent Pupil Defect
D	Distance	RD	Retinal Detachment
DD	Disc Diameter	RE	Refractive Error
DR	Diabetic Retinopathy	RGP	Rigid Gas Permeable
DV	Distance Vision	RHS	Right-Hand Side
EOM	Extraocular Muscle	RP	Retinal Pigmentosa
FFA	Fluorescein Angiography	RPE	Retinal Pigment Epithelium
FH	Family History	PVD	Posterior Vitreous Detachment
Fl	Fluorescein	RX	Prescription
FN	False Negative	S	Without
FP	False Positive	SAC	Seasonal Allergic Conjunctivitis
GP	General Practitioner	SiH	Silicone Hydrogel
H	Horizontal	SN	Superior Nasal
HES	Hospital Eye Services	SO	Superior Oblique
HH	Homonymous Hemianopia	SR	Superior Rectus
HM	Hand Movement	ST	Sight Test
HR	Hypertensive Retinopathy	ST	Superior Temporal
HT	Hypertension	SV	Single Vision
HVID	Horizontal Visible Iris Diameter	Sx	Symptoms
H&S	History and Symptoms	TBUT	Tear Break-up Time
IO	Inferior Oblique	TIA	Transient Ischemic Attack
IOP	Intra Ocular Pressure	UV	Ultraviolet
IR	Inferior Rectus	VA	Visual Acuity
IRMA	Intraretinal microvascular abnormalities	VDU	Visual Display Unit
ISNT	(inferior ≥ superior ≥ nasal ≥ temporal)	VF	Visual Field
IT	Inferior Temporal	VH	Van Herrick
L	Left	WT	Wearing Time
LEE	Last Eye Examination	X	None
		XOP	Exophoria

BIBLIOGRAPHY

1. Alves, M., Miranda, A., Narciso, M., Mieiro, L. and Fonseca, T. (2015). 'Diplopia: A Diagnostic Challenge with Common and Rare Etiologies', American Journal of Case Reports, 16, pp 220-223.
2. American Academy of Ophthalmology. (2022). EyeWiki. Available at: https://eyewiki.org (Accessed 3 October 2022).
3. Anderson, D.R. and Patella, V.M. (1999). Automated Static Perimetry. St. Louis: Mosby.
4. Benjamin, W. and Borish, I. (1998). Borish's Clinical Refraction. Philadelphia: W.B. Saunders, pp.170-172.
5. Bressler, N.M., Bressler, S.B and Fine, S.L. (2006). Retina: Chapter 61. Neovascular (Exudative) Age-Related Macular Degeneration. 4th edn. Mosby: Elsevier, pp 1075-1113
6. Brown, D., Emanuelli, A., Bandello, F., Barranco, J., Figueira, J., Souied, E., Wolf, S., Gupta, V., Ngah, N., Liew, G., Tuli, R., Tadayoni, R., Dhoot, D., Wang, L., Bouillaud, E., Wang, Y., Kovacic, L., Guerard, N. and Garweg, J. (2022). 'KESTREL and KITE: 52-Week Results From Two Phase III Pivotal Trials of Brolucizumab for Diabetic Macular Edema'. American Journal of Ophthalmology, 238, pp 157-172.
7. Clemons, T.E., Milton, R.C., Klein, R., Sedon, J.M. and Ferris, F.L. (2005). 'Risk factors for the incidence of advanced age-related macular degeneration in the Age-Related Eye Disease Study (AREDS): AREDS report no. 19'. Opthalmology, 112(4), pp533-539
8. Denniston A, Murray P. (2006). Oxford Handbook of Ophthalmology. Oxford, United Kingdom: Oxford University Press, pp 276-277.
9. Dinkin, M. (2014). 'Diagnostic approach to diplopia'. Continuum (Minneapolis, Minn.), 20, pp 942–965.
10. Do, D., Nguyen, Q., Boyer, D., Schmidt-Erfurth, U., Brown, D., Vitti, R., Berliner, A., Gao, B., Zeitz, O., Ruckert, R., Schmelter, T., Sandbrink, R. and Heier, J. (2012). 'One-Year Outcomes of the DA VINCI Study of VEGF Trap-Eye in Eyes with Diabetic Macular Edema'. Ophthalmology, 119(8), pp 1658-1665.
11. Elliott, D.B. (2021). Clinical Procedures in Primary Eye Care. 5th edn. Amsterdam: Elsevier.
12. Eskridge, J., Amos, J. and Bartlett, J. (1991). Clinical Procedures in Optometry. Philadelphia: Lippincott.
13. Evans, B.J.W. (2007). Pickwell's Binocular Vision Anomalies. 5th edn, Oxford: Butterworth-Heinemann.
14. Fingeret, M. and Lewis, T.L. (2001). Primary Care of the Glaucomas. New York: McGraw-Hill.
15. Fletcher, E.C. and Chong, N.V. (2008). 'Looking beyond lucentis on the management of macular degeneration', Eye, 22(6), pp.742–750.
16. Fogt, N., Baughman, B.J. and Good. G. (2000). 'The effect of experience on the detection of small eye movements'. Optom Vision Science. 77(12), pp 670-674.
17. Friedman, D. I. (2010). 'Pearls: diplopia'. Seminars in neurology, 30(1), pp 54–65.

18. Grosso, A., Veglio, F., Porta, M., Grignolo, F.M. and Wong, T.Y. (2005). 'Hypertensive retinopathy revisited: some answers, more questions', British Journal of Ophthalmology, pp 89:1646-1654.
19. Guluma, K. (2013). 'Rosen's Emergency Medicine: Concepts and Clinical Practice', Emergency Medicine, pp. 176-183
20. Harrington, D.O. and Drake, M.V. (1990). The Visual Fields: Text and Atlas of Clinical Perimetry.
21. Hitchings, R. A. (2000). Fundamentals of Clinical Ophthalmology: Glaucoma. London: BMJ.
22. Hollands, H., Johnson, D., Brox, A.C., Almeida, D., Simel, D.L. and Sharma, S. (2009). 'Acute-onset floaters and flashes: is this patient at risk for retinal detachment?'. JAMA. 302(20), pp 2243.
23. Hurcomb, P.G., Wolffsohn, J.S. and Napper, G.A. (2001). 'Ocular signs of systemic hypertension: A Review', Ophthalmic and Physiological Optics, 21(6), pp 430–440.
24. Johnson, M., Kass, M.A., Moses, R.A. and Grodzki, W.J. (1978). 'Increased corneal thickness simulating elevated intraocular pressure', Archives of Ophthalmology. 96(4), pp 664-665.
25. Kaur, A. (2022). An Overview of Migraine Management for Optometrists. Available at: https://eyesoneyecare.com/resources/migraine-management-optometry (Accessed 3 October 2022).
26. NHS. (2022). Retinal migraine. Available at: https://www.nhs.uk/conditions/retinal-migraine (Accessed 3 October 2022).
27. Primatesta, P., Brookes, M. and Poulter, N.R. (2001). 'Improved Hypertension Management and Control', Hypertension, 38(4), pp.827– 832.
28. Rosen, E.S., Eustace, P., Thompson, H.S. and Cumming, H.J.K. (1998). Neuro-Ophthalmology. London: Mosby.
29. Rowe, F. (2008). Visual Fields via the Visual Pathway. New York: Blackwell Publishing.
30. Rucker, J. C. and Tomsak, R. L. (2005). 'Binocular diplopia: A practical approach'. The neurologist, 11(2), pp 98–110.
31. Salmon, J. and Kanski, J. (2020). Kanski's clinical ophthalmology: a systematic approach. 9th edn. Edinburgh: Elsevier.
32. Salmon, J.F. and Kanski, J.J. (1996). Glaucoma: a colour manual of diagnosis and treatment. Edinburgh: Butterworth-Heinemann.
33. Schacknow P and Samples J. (2010). The Glaucoma Book: A Practical, Evidence-Based Approach to Patient Care. New York: Springer; pp 399-420
34. Scheiman, M. and Wick, B. (2013). Clinical Management of Binocular Vision: Heterophoric, Accommodative, and Eye Movement Disorders. 4th edn. Philadelphia: Wolters Kluwer health.
35. Seddon, J.M., George, S. and Rosner, B. (2006). 'Cigarette smoking, fish consumption, omega-3 fatty acid intake, and associations with age- related macular degeneration: the US Twin Study of age-related macular degeneration', Archives of Ophthalmology, 124(7), pp 995–1001.
36. St. Kline, L.B., Arnold, A.C., Eggenberger, E., Forozan, R., Golnik, K.C., Rizzo, J.F. and Shaw, H.E., (2007). 'Basic & Clinical Science Course: Neuro-

Ophthalmology Section 5 2007- 2008', American Academy of Ophthalmology. Louis: The C.V. Mosby Comp.
37. Szatmáry, G. (2002). 'Can Swedish interactive thresholding algorithm fast perimetry be used as an alternative to Goldmann perimetry in neuro-ophthalmic practice?', Archives of Ophthalmology, 120(9), pp. 1162. DOI: 10.1097/00041327-20030300-00017.
38. The Age-Related Eye Disease Study Research Group. (2001). 'A randomized, placebo-controlled, clinical trial of high-dose supplementation with vitamins C and E, beta carotene, and zinc for age- related macular degeneration and vision loss', Archives of ophthalmology, 119(10), pp 1417-1436.
39. The College of Optometrists. (2022). Annex 4 Urgency of referrals table. Available at: https://www.college-optometrists.org/clinical-guidance/guidance/guidance-annexes/annex-4-urgency-of-referrals-table (Accessed 3 October 2022).
40. Wall, M., Punke, S.G., Stickney, T.L., Brito, C.F., Witbrow, K.R. and Kardon, R.H. (2001) 'SITA Standard in optic neuropathies and hemianopias: A comparison with Full Threshold testing', Investigative Ophthalmology & Visual Science, 42(2), pp 528-537.
41. Walsh, T. J. (1997). Neuro- Ophthalmology Clinical Signs and Symptoms. 3rd edn. Philadelphia: Lea & Febiger
42. Wolffsohn, J.S., Napper, G., Ho, S., Jaworski, A, and Pollard, T. (2001). 'Improving the description of the retinal vasculature and patient history taking for monitoring systemic hypertension', Ophthalmic and Physiological Optics, 21(6), pp.441–449. DOI: 10.1046/j.1475-1313.2001.00616.x

ABOUT THE AUTHOR

Founded by Tahiba Begum, Optometry 101 focuses on support and guidance for students and Optometrists.
Our principal aim is to provide a clear understanding of Optometry in everyday practice.

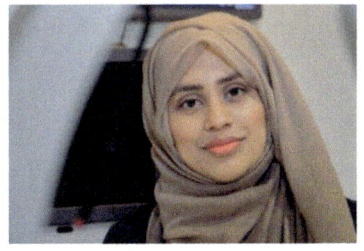

Tahiba Begum is a qualified Optometrist with over ten years of experience in her respective field. She has worked in multiple High Street chains where she completed her pre-registration, after which she successfully progressed as a supervisor and tutor within the industry. Tahiba has aided many students with their training who have qualified as successful Optometrists.

Born in Rochdale, a small town in Greater Manchester, Tahiba successfully obtained the highest GCSE grades in her cohort, which included 8A*s and 5As, withstanding Rochdale's challenging education system. She then progressed to Oldham Sixth Form College and finally completed her BSc in Optometry at Bradford University. Following her residency at Specsavers, Tahiba relocated to London, where she advanced her experience and continues to work as a locum Optometrist in several different optical branches.

She was fortunate to meet many Optometrists and healthcare professionals, each adding valuable insight to her experience. Following on, Tahiba was blessed with two children who came with their challenges, new experiences and put a unique perspective on life. She took a 3-year maternity break to focus primarily on her children. When it was time to return, the overwhelming feeling of returning to work was unexpected. This led to an awe-struck moment of inspiration, and as such, Optometry 101 came to fruition.

"Most ocular pathology books are designed with the Ophthalmologists in mind. Sourcing relevant information can take time; this can become extremely difficult in a busy workplace with a tight schedule. A book at hand, catered towards the Optometrist, with practical guidelines to use in the testing room, will make a difference to the job. Designed with this purpose, Optometry 101 will provide ease to the Optometrist in completing their job to the best of their ability."